Carb-Conscious LIVING

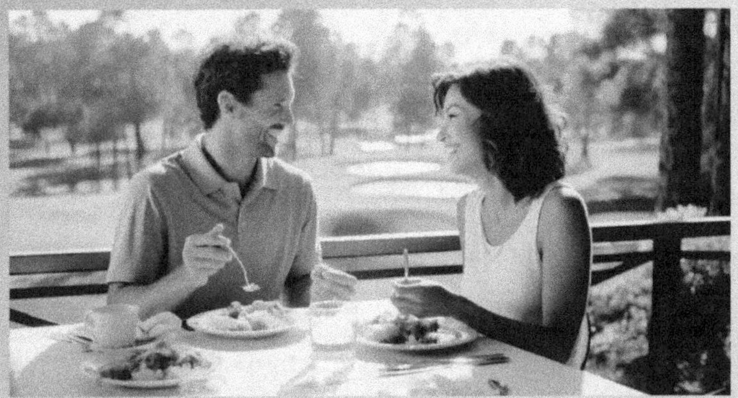

A Guide to Maintaining a Healthy Lifestyle on a Low-Carb Diet

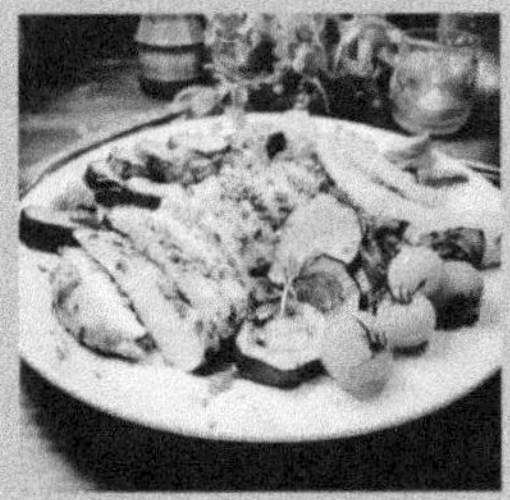
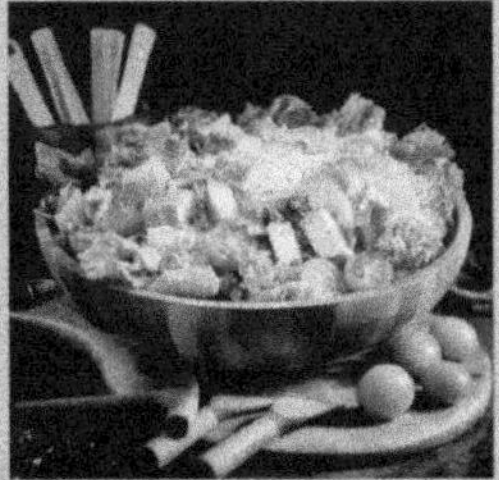
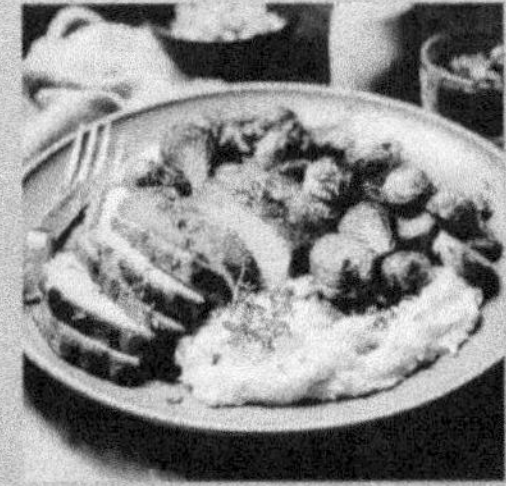

by Mike Cunningham

Contents

Preface

For most of my life I have been fighting my own "Battle of the Bulge." As a teenager I was always the largest kid in my class and by eighth grade I had topped 200 pounds. Fortunately, I was also one of the tallest and have spent most of my adult life at 6' 2", Like so many of us, I have yoyo dieted for years, in my 30's I lost nearly 100 pounds with Weight Watchers but found the extra pounds later in many bags of potato chips and snacks. In my 50's I discovered The South Beach Diet, a low-carb program that helped me lose 120 pounds. Now 20 years later I have managed to keep most of the weight off, but it's still a battle that I too often lose.

I don't know if it's a scientific fact but I think it's harder to lose weight through dieting as we age. I know from experience that men in general lose weight faster than women. Now at age 75 I have succumbed to the lure of snacking again. I think our current retired lifestyle has an influence on the way I eat. I try to stay active with golf and aqua aerobics at least twice each week and that bit of exercise is probably helping me maintain.

We can always find an excuse to eat: the Holidays (I'll cut back right after New Year's Day), travel and cruising (what will one more slice of delicious cruise pie matter), and the most dangerous, snacking while watching television (can't watch football without some ice cream and potato chips). I'm sharing this book with you dear reader, because I think it's time for me to find some motivation to get back on the low-carb wagon, and by presenting this information to you, I hope it will help guide and inspire you and encourage me to return to the world of low-carb eating....ahhh Ketosis here we come!

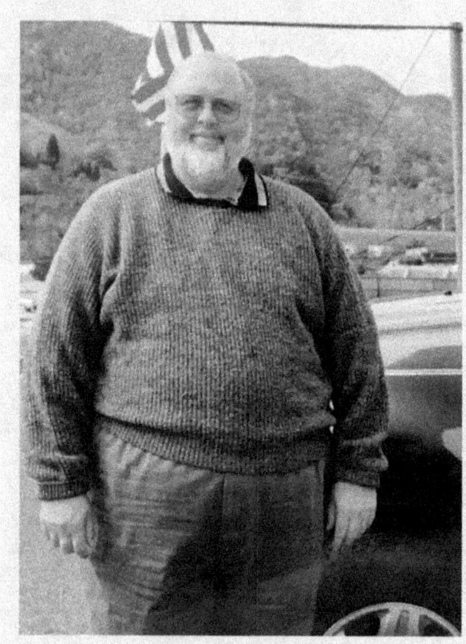
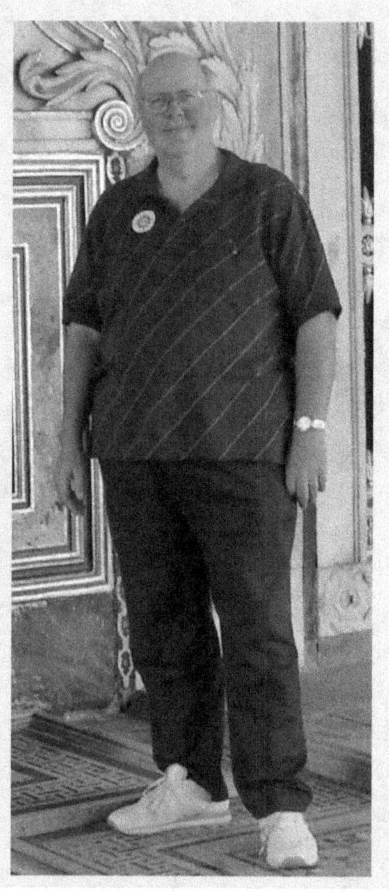

Introduction

Hello and welcome to "Carb-Conscious Living: A Guide to Maintaining a Healthy Lifestyle on a Low-Carb Diet." Navigating through numerous dietary choices can be challenging, each with its own intricacies. Achieving well-being is both admirable and complex. This book aims to be your informative companion on the journey to a healthier life, providing practical insights, actionable strategies, and a wealth of information to help you embrace a low-carb lifestyle.

As we dive into the upcoming sections, we aim to present a story that goes beyond typical diet information. We're not just talking about managing weight; our main goal is to encourage a lasting, balanced approach to nutrition and overall well-being. Whether you're new to exploring the low-carb lifestyle or looking for insightful perspectives as someone experienced in this approach, this guide is carefully crafted to meet you where you are in your journey.

In this introduction, we lay the foundation by exploring the basics of low-carb living, explaining the important role of maintaining a healthy lifestyle and outlining the specific goals of this book as a comprehensive resource. We invite you to join us on a transformative intellectual journey that blends the science of nutrition, mindful eating, the benefits of physical activity, and the skill needed to shape a life aligned with your health goals..

In the upcoming chapters, we'll explore the detailed world of low-carb diets, break down the complexities of creating balanced meal plans, and provide practical advice on smoothly integrating these changes into your daily routine. Apart from focusing on food choices, we'll delve into the essential role of physical activity, the connection between mindful eating and emotional well-being, and present strategies for overcoming the inevitable challenges that come with this transformative journey.

Whether you're aiming for weight management, improved blood sugar control, increased energy levels, or an overall approach to health and vitality, "Carb Conscious Living" is ready to be your steadfast guide. Embrace the valuable insights found in these pages, incorporate the knowledge into your daily habits, and look forward to the positive transformation that stems from making informed decisions.

Overview: Embracing the Low-Carb Lifestyle within Carb Conscious Living

The low-carb lifestyle, as outlined by Carb-Conscious Living, represents a mindful and purposeful approach to nutrition aimed at improving health. At its core, this lifestyle emphasizes a careful decrease in carbohydrate consumption, recognizing the significant impact of dietary choices on vital factors like weight, blood sugar, and overall metabolic health.

This method is based on the idea that the amount and type of carbohydrates you eat can have a notable effect on your overall health. Choosing a low-carb lifestyle means deliberately shaping your diet in a thoughtful and nuanced way, using nutrition to enhance different aspects of your well-being.

Weight management, a cornerstone of this lifestyle, is addressed through the calculated limitation of carbohydrate intake. Recognizing that excessive carb consumption can contribute to weight gain, the low-carb approach provides a structured framework for individuals seeking to achieve and maintain a healthy weight.

Furthermore, intentionally cutting down on carbohydrates is in line with controlling blood sugar levels. When individuals moderate their consumption of sugars and refined carbohydrates, it helps reduce the chances of blood glucose fluctuations, fostering more consistent energy levels and maintaining metabolic stability.

This way of life also emphasizes its dedication to overall metabolic health, highlighting the relationship between dietary choices and physical well-being. When individuals choose nutrient-dense, low-carb foods, they are better able to nurture their metabolism, promoting a state of equilibrium and vitality.

In essence, the low-carb lifestyle, as part of Carbo-Conscious Living, embodies a comprehensive and knowledgeable approach to nutrition. Intentionally reducing carbohydrate intake, enables individuals to make thoughtful choices that positively impact weight management, blood sugar regulation, and overall metabolic health, paving the way towards optimal well-being.

Foundations of Low-Carb Living:

The core tenets of Low-Carb Living are built on a key principle—promoting a purposeful decrease in the intake of carbohydrates, particularly by restricting refined sugars and starches. This dietary strategy is grounded in a thorough comprehension that high levels of carbohydrate consumption may lead to unfavorable outcomes like fluctuations in blood sugar, insulin resistance, and consequent weight gain. Through emphasizing moderation in carbohydrate intake, this lifestyle seeks to empower individuals to gain improved control over their blood sugar levels, thereby promoting overall metabolic health.

At the heart of this philosophy is the understanding that consuming too many refined sugars and starches can result in unfavorable effects on the body. These effects include quick increases and decreases in blood sugar levels, which, over time, might contribute to the onset of insulin resistance—a state where the body's cells become less responsive to the hormone insulin. This resistance can subsequently lead to challenges in properly regulating blood sugar, posing a threat to metabolic health.

Furthermore, the link between consuming too many carbohydrates and gaining weight is a fundamental aspect of the low-carb lifestyle. The reasoning is that when the body gets an excess of carbohydrates, particularly from refined sugars and starches, it might store the extra energy as fat. Through moderating carbohydrate intake, individuals aim to better control their weight and decrease the chances of accumulating surplus body fat.

Essentially, the principles of Low-Carb Living promote a thoughtful and intentional way of making dietary decisions, particularly regarding carbohydrates. This lifestyle underscores the importance of limiting refined sugars and starches to minimize the potential risks linked to disruptions in blood sugar, insulin resistance, and weight gain. By adopting this approach, individuals actively work towards improving blood sugar regulation and enhancing their overall metabolic health. This aligns with the overarching objective of cultivating a balanced and sustainable approach to well-being.

Strategic Carbohydrate Choices:

Choosing Carbohydrates wisely is a crucial element of the Carbo-Conscious Living philosophy, urging a thoughtful approach to picking carbohydrate sources. In this context, the focus is on making intentional choices that adhere to the principles of health and nutrition. While limiting refined carbohydrates and sugars, the emphasis is on including nutrient-dense, fiber-rich carbohydrates, such as vegetables, fruits, and whole grains.

This thoughtful approach demonstrates a dedication to sustaining a balanced and nutritionally beneficial diet, even with a decrease in carbohydrate consumption. Vegetables, fruits, and whole grains are chosen for their natural abundance of essential vitamins, minerals, and dietary fiber. These elements not only enhance the overall nutritional content of the diet but also play a vital role in promoting digestive health, satisfaction, and a consistent release of energy.

Through the deliberate selection of these particular carbohydrate sources, individuals engaging in Carbo-Conscious Living find a harmony between controlling their overall carbohydrate intake and guaranteeing the body obtains essential nutrients. The incorporation of fiber, specifically, supports digestive regulation and fosters a sense of fullness, which plays a crucial role in managing overall calorie consumption.

The intentional selection of these carbohydrate options is in line with the primary objective of Carbo-Conscious Living—to enhance health without sacrificing vital nutrients. This strategy acknowledges that not all carbohydrates are the same, and by choosing sources that provide nutritional benefits, individuals can navigate the intricacies of dietary decisions more effectively.

In conclusion, the philosophy of Carbo-Conscious Living encourages individuals to make deliberate and careful choices when it comes to carbohydrates. This involves minimizing refined carbohydrates and sugars while embracing nutrient-dense and fiber-rich options. By doing so, individuals can find a balance between controlling their carbohydrate intake and maintaining a diet that supports their overall health and well-being.

Balanced Macronutrient Ratios:

In the Carbo-Conscious Living philosophy, maintaining Balanced Macronutrient Ratios is a key principle. This highlights the significance of achieving a harmonious balance among the three primary macronutrients in one's diet. While this lifestyle involves purposefully limiting carbohydrate intake, it equally stresses the intentional inclusion of an adequate amount of protein and healthy fats in the overall dietary approach.

This thoughtful approach acknowledges the unique roles that each macronutrient plays in sustaining bodily functions and promoting overall health. Proteins, crucial for maintaining muscles, facilitating repair, and supporting metabolic processes, are included in sufficient amounts to uphold the body's structural integrity and ensure optimal function. Moreover, intentionally including healthy fats from sources like avocados, nuts, and olive oil serves multiple functions. Apart from being a concentrated energy source, these fats play a role in hormone production, aiding nutrient absorption, and maintaining cellular health.

In Carbo-Conscious Living, the intentional reduction of carbohydrates is paired with a mindful approach to avoid extremes, promoting a balanced intake of all three macronutrients. This approach not only guards against potential nutrient deficiencies but also enhances satiety, the feeling of fullness and satisfaction after meals. Striking this balance fosters a sustainable and nourishing approach to nutrition, ensuring that individuals can adhere to their dietary choices over the long term.

Moreover, in adhering to balanced macronutrient ratios, Carbo-Conscious Living aims to reject the idea of condemning any particular macronutrient category. Instead, it encourages a comprehensive comprehension of the body's nutritional requirements, recognizing that a well-rounded combination of carbohydrates, proteins, and fats is vital for attaining optimal health and functionality.

In conclusion, following Balanced Macronutrient Ratios in Carbo-Conscious Living represents a thoughtful and comprehensive dietary approach. By controlling carbohydrate intake and deliberately including sufficient protein and healthy fats, individuals can maintain a nutritional balance that supports feelings of fullness and offers the necessary components for overall health and optimal bodily function.

Meal Planning and Preparation:

Meal Planning and Preparation play a pivotal role in the philosophy of Carbo-Conscious Living, highlighting the importance of intentional and considerate approaches to dietary decisions. This aspect of the lifestyle entails carefully creating well-balanced and gratifying meals customized to meet individual health objectives. By adhering to the principles of whole, minimally processed foods and incorporating portion control, individuals can navigate their low-carb journey with practicality and ease.

The purposeful aspect of meal planning within Carbo-Conscious Living entails a systematic evaluation of the nutritional elements in every meal. It involves the meticulous selection of whole foods, including lean proteins, vibrant vegetables, and nutrient-rich sources of healthy fats. This methodology guarantees that meals not only align with low-carb principles but also deliver a comprehensive range of essential vitamins, minerals, and other crucial nutrients.

Controlling portion sizes becomes a pivotal tactic in this undertaking, empowering individuals to regulate calorie intake and uphold a balanced macronutrient composition. By comprehending and managing the amounts of each food group, individuals can achieve a harmonious equilibrium in line with their dietary goals, be it centered around weight management, blood sugar control, or overall metabolic health.

Moreover, the focus on meal preparation underscores the practicality of Carbo-Conscious Living. By dedicating time to plan and prepare meals in advance, individuals streamline their daily routines and diminish dependence on convenient or processed foods. This not only elevates the nutritional value of the diet but also nurtures a sustainable and enduring commitment to the low-carb lifestyle.

Essentially, the proactive and purposeful approach to nutrition embedded in Meal Planning and Preparation within Carbo-Conscious Living highlights the crafting of well-balanced, satisfying meals. This approach, emphasizing whole foods and portion control, empowers individuals to navigate their low-carb journey with practicality, fostering both the effectiveness and sustainability of their dietary choices.

Physical Activity Integration:

Physical Activity Integration is a core tenet of the Carbo-Conscious Living philosophy, recognizing the interconnectedness of nutrition and exercise in achieving holistic well-being. Beyond its primary emphasis on dietary choices, this lifestyle underscores the symbiotic relationship between nutrition and physical activity. Regular exercise is not considered optional but is viewed as an integral and complementary element of the Carbo-Conscious Living paradigm. It plays a crucial role in weight management, enhancing insulin sensitivity, and contributing to overall well-being.

Understanding the synergistic relationship between nutrition and physical activity emphasizes the holistic approach inherent in Carbo-Conscious Living. Regular exercise is advocated not only for its established benefits in burning calories and managing weight but also for its profound impact on metabolic health. Consistent physical activity is linked to heightened insulin sensitivity, enabling the body to regulate blood sugar levels more effectively. This is especially pertinent in the context of a low-carb lifestyle, where optimizing blood sugar control is a central goal.

Furthermore, physical activity is acknowledged as a significant contributor to overall well-being. In addition to its direct impact on body composition and metabolic function, exercise has been associated with improved mood, enhanced cognitive function, and a decreased risk of various chronic diseases. This comprehensive viewpoint aligns with the broader objective of Carbo-Conscious Living, aiming to advocate not only specific dietary practices but also a holistic lifestyle conducive to optimal health.

Promoting regular exercise within the framework of Carbo-Conscious Living extends beyond the conventional view of physical activity as a way to burn calories. It signifies an awareness that an active lifestyle is intricately connected to overall health. By incorporating physical activity into daily routines, individuals not only boost the effectiveness of their low-carb approach but also nurture a sustainable and holistic foundation for well-being.

In conclusion, the incorporation of Physical Activity within Carbo-Conscious Living demonstrates a nuanced comprehension of the interconnection between nutrition and exercise. Acknowledging exercise as a vital element, this lifestyle advocates for weight management, enhanced insulin sensitivity, and overall well-being, in harmony with its dedication to a comprehensive and sustainable approach to health.

Mindful Eating and Emotional Well-Being:

Mindful Eating and Emotional Well-Being play crucial roles in the structure of Carbo-Conscious Living, emphasizing the deep link between eating habits and emotional health. Central to this lifestyle is the adoption of mindful eating—a purposeful method involving heightened awareness of food choices, relishing meals, and tuning into the body's hunger and fullness signals.

Practicing mindful eating in Carbo-Conscious Living goes beyond choosing low-carb foods—it involves a deliberate and present-focused involvement with the entire eating experience. This encompasses appreciating the textures, flavors, and aromas of each meal, creating a profound connection with the act of nourishment. By slowing down the eating process and staying fully engaged, individuals are prompted to make informed and gratifying food choices, fostering a sense of satisfaction that transcends mere nutritional value.

In addition to the physical aspects of eating, Carbo-Conscious Living acknowledges and addresses the emotional dimensions associated with food consumption. The lifestyle recognizes that individuals may resort to food as a means of coping with stress or emotional triggers. Accordingly, it provides strategies to navigate these emotional aspects without turning to unhealthy dietary habits. By fostering an increased awareness of emotional eating patterns, individuals can cultivate alternative coping mechanisms that enhance emotional well-being while staying true to their commitment to a low-carb lifestyle.

This approach aligns with the overarching objective of Carbo-Conscious Living—to establish a sustainable and holistic relationship with food. By integrating mindful eating practices and addressing emotional well-being, individuals not only optimize their nutritional choices but also cultivate a positive and balanced attitude toward food. This, in turn, contributes to a more comprehensive sense of well-being that extends beyond physical health to encompass emotional resilience and self-awareness.

In summary, Mindful Eating and Emotional Well-Being are integral components of Carbo-Conscious Living. By promoting a mindful approach to food choices and addressing emotional aspects of eating, this lifestyle not only enhances the effectiveness of a low-carb diet but also fosters a holistic and sustainable foundation for overall health and well-being.

Sustainability and Long-Term Success:

Sustainability and Long-Term Success are fundamental principles of the Carbo-Conscious Living philosophy, positioning it not as a temporary diet but as a lasting lifestyle choice. This approach prioritizes the cultivation of a sustainable and enduring commitment to health and wellness. By imparting a comprehensive understanding of nutritional principles, offering practical meal planning tips, and providing strategies for overcoming challenges, Carbo-Conscious Living empowers individuals to achieve and maintain their health goals over the long term.

The distinctive quality of Carbo-Conscious Living lies in its commitment to surpassing the temporary nature often linked with various dietary trends. Instead of enforcing strict rules, it provides a profound understanding of nutritional concepts, empowering individuals to make informed and mindful choices. This knowledge serves as the basis for a sustainable approach to dietary habits—one that can adapt to different lifestyles and be maintained throughout an individual's journey toward well-being.

Practical meal planning is a fundamental aspect of maintaining sustainability within Carbo-Conscious Living. The philosophy acknowledges the necessity of translating nutritional principles into practical, real-world applications. By providing tips and guidance on planning and preparing meals in alignment with the low-carb lifestyle, individuals gain the necessary tools to seamlessly integrate this approach into their daily lives. This not only amplifies the effectiveness of the lifestyle but also nurtures a sense of practicality and ease in its application.

Tackling challenges represents a crucial aspect of Carbo-Conscious Living's dedication to long-term success. By recognizing potential obstacles and offering strategies to overcome them, the lifestyle empowers individuals with the resilience and adaptability essential for consistent adherence. This forward-looking perspective ensures that challenges are not perceived as insurmountable barriers but rather as opportunities for personal growth and refinement within one's health journey.

At its core, Carbo-Conscious Living embodies a comprehensive and knowledgeable approach to nutrition. Promoting mindful decision-making and equipping individuals with practical tools for implementation, nurtures optimal health, balanced well-being, and enduring vitality. Positioned as a lifestyle choice rather than a passing trend, Carbo-Conscious Living serves as a testament to a sustained dedication to health and wellness over the long term.

Maintaining a Healthy Lifestyle on a Low-Carb Diet: A Vital Balancing Act

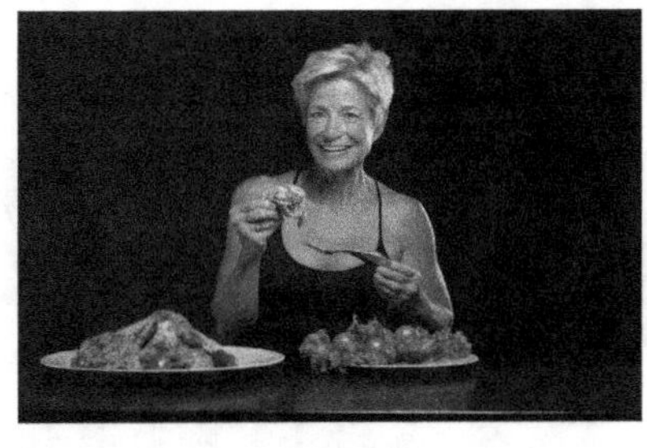

In the quest for optimal health, the significance of embracing a healthy lifestyle alongside a low-carb diet cannot be emphasized enough. A low-carb lifestyle, marked by a deliberate reduction in carbohydrate intake, not only provides various health advantages but truly reveals its transformative power when combined with a holistic approach to well-being.

Weight Management:

Managing weight takes on a crucial role as a primary incentive for adopting a low-carb lifestyle, showcasing a purposeful and calculated strategy for attaining and maintaining a healthy body weight. This lifestyle decision is based on the concept of controlling carbohydrate intake, especially by limiting refined sugars and starches. The objective is to regulate caloric

consumption, enabling weight loss and, significantly, establishing enduring habits that support ongoing weight management.

Purposefully limiting carbohydrate intake, particularly refined carbs, is
grounded in the idea that excessive consumption of carbs can be a factor in
weight gain. Refined sugars and starches, commonly found in numerous
processed foods, can cause spikes in blood sugar levels, leading the body to
store surplus energy as fat. Embracing a low-carb strategy seeks to break
this cycle, prompting the body to utilize stored fat for energy and, as a
result, fostering weight loss.

Looking beyond the primary objective of losing extra weight, the importance of weight management in the context of the low-carb lifestyle
involves fostering habits that are sustainable. In contrast to short-term
diets that may provide temporary results, the emphasis is placed on establishing lasting dietary practices that can be upheld over an extended
period. Prioritizing sustainability not only aids in weight loss endeavors
but also encourages the cultivation of a healthy and balanced connection
with food.

The low-carb lifestyle recognizes that effective weight management extends beyond simple restriction; it requires thoughtful and informed dietary decision-making. Through the inclusion of nutrient-dense foods and
a focus on a well-balanced macronutrient profile, individuals can ade-
quately nourish their bodies while actively pursuing their weight management objectives. This comprehensive approach aligns with the core philosophy of Carbo-Conscious Living, emphasizing long-term well-being over
short-term solutions.

Blood Sugar Control:

Maintaining control over blood sugar levels is a key advantage of adopting
a low-carb diet, especially for those dealing with conditions like diabetes
or insulin resistance. In this context, a low-carb dietary approach plays a
crucial role in stabilizing blood sugar levels, providing a strategic method
to address the challenges linked to glucose regulation.

The core idea behind the low-carb diet is deliberately cutting down on
the intake of carbohydrates, with a particular emphasis on minimizing

the consumption of refined sugars and starches. This approach enables individuals to effectively handle the fluctuations in blood glucose levels often triggered by high-carbohydrate foods. This careful control is a crucial strategy to improve insulin sensitivity, playing a significant role in managing conditions like diabetes and insulin resistance.

Insulin sensitivity denotes how effectively the body responds to insulin, the hormone responsible for managing blood sugar levels. Embracing a low-carb diet aims to decrease the reliance on insulin, empowering the body to regulate blood glucose levels more effectively. This holds particular importance for individuals with diabetes, where maintaining stable blood sugar levels is crucial for minimizing the risk of complications associated with the condition.

Stabilizing blood sugar levels by adopting a low-carb approach plays a crucial role in enhancing overall metabolic health. Maintaining consistent and controlled blood sugar levels supports the body's regulatory mechanisms, fostering a balanced state that goes beyond glucose regulation. This, in turn, can positively impact various facets of metabolic function, including weight management and cardiovascular health.

The precise management of blood sugar levels, attained through a low-carb diet, resonates with the overarching principles of Carbo-Conscious Living. Through conscious decisions to restrict carbohydrate intake and prioritize nutrient-dense alternatives, individuals not only address immediate concerns regarding blood sugar control but also cultivate a sustainable and holistic approach to metabolic health.

Increased Energy Levels:

Embracing a well-structured low-carb diet has the potential to bring about a significant boost in energy levels. This results in a sustainable source of vitality, surpassing the fleeting spikes and crashes typically linked to high-carbohydrate meals. The positive influence on energy is credited to the intentional inclusion of nutrient-dense, whole foods, which support a consistent release of energy throughout the day.

A key factor contributing to the success of a low-carb diet is the focus on nutrient-dense options, such as lean proteins, healthy fats, and fibrous vegetables. These foods, abundant in essential vitamins and minerals, furnish the body with a steady and well-rounded supply of nutrients. In contrast to high-carbohydrate meals that can result in abrupt spikes and subsequent declines in blood sugar levels, the nutrient-dense nature of a low-carb diet encourages a more consistent and prolonged release of energy.

By steering clear of the ups and downs linked to blood sugar changes, individuals adhering to a low-carb diet can lessen the energy crashes frequently experienced after consuming high-carbohydrate meals. This enduring energy is advantageous not only for physical activities but also for cognitive abilities and mental clarity. Evading fluctuations in energy levels assist in sustaining focus and alertness throughout the day, fostering an overall sense of well-being.

Relying on whole foods in a low-carb diet is in harmony with the principles of Carbo-Conscious Living, underscoring the significance of making thoughtful and informed dietary choices. This method not only boosts energy levels but also nurtures a comprehensive comprehension of nutrition, urging individuals to prioritize foods that enhance both physical and mental vitality.

Essentially, the rise in sustained energy levels resulting from a well-structured low-carb diet represents a departure from the unpredictable energy fluctuations linked to high-carbohydrate meals. This intentional dietary strategy, focusing on nutrient-dense foods, not only improves physical performance but also supports cognitive function and mental clarity, in line with the overarching principles of Carbo-Conscious Living.

Cardiovascular Health:

A low-carb lifestyle, especially when emphasizing the inclusion of healthy fats and lean proteins, has been associated with significant enhancements in cardiovascular health. This dietary strategy entails purposefully decreasing the intake of processed carbohydrates and trans fats, providing a strategic approach to positively impact lipid profiles, alleviate inflammation, and contribute to a healthier heart. These diverse advantages not only promote longevity but also cultivate overall cardiovascular well-being.

At the heart of the cardiovascular advantages linked to a low-carb lifestyle is the focus on including healthy fats and lean proteins. Healthy fats, sourced from items like avocados, nuts, and olive oil, promote a favorable lipid profile by elevating levels of high-density lipoprotein (HDL or "good" cholesterol) and lowering levels of low-density lipoprotein (LDL or "bad" cholesterol). Striking this balance is vital for preserving arterial health and diminishing the risk of atherosclerosis.

At the same time, minimizing the consumption of processed carbohydrates aids in reducing the risk of elevated triglyceride levels, a significant factor in lipid profiles. Processed carbohydrates, commonly present in sugary and refined foods, can lead to higher triglycerides, associated with an increased risk of cardiovascular problems. Through moderating carbohydrate intake, individuals adhering to a low-carb lifestyle strive to optimize their lipid profiles and promote heart health.

In addition to impacting lipid profiles, a low-carb lifestyle tackles inflammation, a recognized contributor to cardiovascular diseases. By reducing the intake of trans fats, commonly present in processed and fried foods, individuals can decrease systemic inflammation. This promotes healthier blood vessels and lowers the risk of cardiovascular events.

The collective impact of these dietary choices goes beyond immediate benefits, contributing to longevity and overall cardiovascular well-being. A low-carb lifestyle, particularly when emphasizing healthy fats and lean proteins, mirrors the principles of Carbo-Conscious Living, providing a comprehensive approach to fostering heart health.

Cognitive Benefits:

Recent studies have highlighted a potential connection between a low-carb diet and cognitive advantages, revealing the complex interplay between dietary decisions and cognitive function. This nutritional strategy, marked by the control of blood sugar swings and the support of a consistent energy supply to the brain, shows the potential to improve cognitive abilities and potentially lowering the risk of neurodegenerative conditions.

A key element in the cognitive advantages linked to a low-carb diet is its influence on blood sugar levels. By decreasing the consumption of carbohydrates, especially those swiftly processed that result in quick spikes in blood glucose, individuals can steer clear of the subsequent drops commonly associated with high-carb meals. This stabilization of blood sugar levels is crucial for sustaining cognitive function, as the brain heavily depends on a steady and regulated supply of glucose for optimal performance.

Moreover, the steady and lasting energy supplied by a low-carb diet is believed to have a positive impact on cognitive abilities. Steering clear of the fluctuations in energy commonly associated with high-carbohydrate meals may play a role in enhancing focus, concentration, and mental clarity. Consequently, this could have implications for tasks that demand cognitive engagement, including problem-solving, memory retention, and overall cognitive performance.

While the precise ways in which a low-carb diet enhances cognitive function are still under investigation, there is increasing curiosity about its ability to lower the risk of neurodegenerative conditions. Certain studies propose that the metabolic and anti-inflammatory impacts of a low-carb lifestyle might create a neuroprotective environment, potentially diminishing the chances of cognitive decline linked to aging.

In summary, the evolving research on cognitive advantages linked to a low-carb diet highlights the complex connection between dietary decisions and brain health. This dietary approach, which minimizes blood sugar swings and ensures a consistent energy supply to the brain, might enhance cognitive performance and potentially provide protective effects against neurodegenerative conditions. As our knowledge of this relationship develops, the potential implications for cognitive health in the context of a low-carb lifestyle are gaining increased attention.

Holistic Well-Being:

In the realm of a low-carb diet, holistic well-being goes beyond concentrating solely on specific health indicators. It acknowledges the interdependence of various lifestyle factors, enhancing the advantages of the low-carb approach. Holistic well-being underscores the importance of not only dietary aspects but also regular physical activity, proper hydration, ample sleep, and effective stress management. These elements collectively form a comprehensive health strategy.

A key principle of holistic well-being is understanding that health is a complex concept shaped by both dietary and lifestyle decisions. While the low-carb diet tackles particular aspects like weight management and blood sugar control, incorporating additional lifestyle factors ensures a more comprehensive and balanced approach to health.

Regular physical activity plays a crucial role in holistic well-being, aiding in physical fitness and weight management while also enhancing cardiovascular health, muscle strength, and mental well-being. The harmonious balance achieved by combining a low-carb diet with regular exercise contributes to overall vitality.

Sufficient hydration is a crucial element of holistic well-being. Proper hydration supports the metabolic processes linked to a low-carb diet and enhances cognitive function, joint health, and overall bodily function. Integrating mindful hydration practices with a low-carb approach helps the body function optimally.

Adequate sleep is acknowledged as a crucial factor in holistic well-being. Quality sleep is linked to improved immune function, cognitive performance, and emotional resilience. When combined with a low-carb lifestyle, sufficient sleep establishes a synergistic relationship, boosting the body's ability to recover and rejuvenate.

Effective stress management completes the elements of holistic well-being. Chronic stress can influence various aspects of health, including inflammation, hormone balance, and mental well-being. By integrating stress-reducing practices like mindfulness, meditation, or relaxation techniques with a low-carb diet, individuals establish a comprehensive approach that addresses both the physical and mental aspects of well-being.

Sustainability and Long-Term Success:

Creating a lasting and successful approach to health, especially when embracing a low-carb diet, relies on sustainability and long-term commitment. While the positive effects of the diet may be noticeable in the short run, their lasting impact is optimized when incorporated into a lifestyle that is both enduring and comprehensive. This enduring commitment is essential for navigating the challenges of daily life, adhering to dietary choices in various social settings, and developing healthy habits that can be sustained throughout a lifetime.

Recognizing the importance of sustainability involves understanding that health is an ongoing journey, and embracing a low-carb diet is just one aspect of this broader effort. While the diet may provide noticeable and quick advantages, maintaining its success requires a comprehensive approach that goes beyond dietary factors.

A sustainable lifestyle, in this context, involves making choices that support health goals while considering the realities of everyday life. It acknowledges that people encounter different social settings, work obligations, and personal commitments that can affect their adherence to a specific diet. Integrating a low-carb approach into the broader context of a healthy lifestyle provides flexibility and adaptability, enabling individuals to make health-conscious choices in various situations.

Moreover, maintaining healthy habits depends on having a positive and balanced relationship with food. By developing nutrition knowledge, encouraging mindful eating habits, and including enjoyable and satisfying meals, individuals are more likely to stick to their commitment to a low-carb lifestyle in the long run.

Taking a holistic approach to well-being, which involves not just dietary choices but also physical activity, hydration, sleep, and stress management, strengthens the sustainability of healthy habits. This comprehensive strategy provides individuals with the tools to manage various aspects of their well-being, establishing a robust foundation for long-term success.

In essence, sustainability and long-term success within a low-carb lifestyle reflect a dedication to health as an ongoing journey. Embracing a holistic approach that takes into account different aspects of well-being allows individuals to navigate life's challenges, stick to dietary choices in various settings, and develop healthful habits that endure. This persistent commitment to health emphasizes the significance of incorporating a low-carb diet into a wider framework of sustainable lifestyle practices.

In conclusion, combining a low-carb diet with a holistic approach to a healthy lifestyle proves to be a potent strategy for attaining and sustaining optimal well-being. Beyond the evident health advantages, this collaboration nurtures a balanced and lasting way of life, enabling individuals not only to reshape their bodies but also to foster enduring habits that enhance vitality, resilience, and a fulfilling life.

The Journey to Optimal Health

The purpose of "Carbo-Conscious Living: A Guide to Maintaining a Healthy Lifestyle on a Low-Carb Diet" is multifaceted, aiming to empower individuals in their journey towards optimal health and well-being within the context of a low-carb lifestyle. This book is designed with the following key objectives in mind:

Comprehensive Understanding:

The goal of this book is to provide readers with a thorough grasp of the principles and intricacies involved in embracing a low-carb lifestyle. Through careful exploration, the book aims to clarify the scientific foundations of low-carb diets, articulate their advantages, and thoughtfully dispel any potential misconceptions. The ultimate objective is to equip individuals with the knowledge needed to make well-informed decisions about their dietary preferences, cultivating a deeper and more nuanced understanding of the low-carb lifestyle.

The essence of this book lies in its dedication to clarity and accuracy when explaining the scientific basis of low-carb diets. It explores the physiological and metabolic dimensions, offering readers insights into how the body reacts to a decrease in carbohydrate intake. Through the clarification of the underlying science, the book seeks to unravel the mechanisms that underpin the effectiveness of a low-carb lifestyle, providing readers with a strong foundation to inform their dietary choices.

Beyond deciphering the science, this book systematically outlines the tangible advantages linked to embracing a low-carb approach. Covering areas such as weight management, blood sugar control, cognitive benefits, and cardiovascular health, it provides readers with a holistic perspective on the positive outcomes that can arise from adopting a low-carb lifestyle.

Acknowledging the potential for misinformation to cloud public perception, this book takes on the responsibility of dispelling common misconceptions surrounding low-carb diets. By addressing prevalent myths and providing evidence-based insights, it aims to equip readers with the discernment needed to navigate the sometimes confusing landscape of dietary information.

Beyond presenting facts, the book aspires to cultivate a genuine understanding of the principles and nuances of a low-carb lifestyle. Through a well-rounded exploration that encompasses both the scientific foundations and practical benefits, it seeks to empower individuals to make thoughtful and informed choices about their dietary habits. In doing so, it becomes a valuable resource for those looking to embrace a low-carb lifestyle with a comprehensive understanding that goes beyond surface-level information.

Practical Guidance:

Understanding the theoretical foundations of a low-carb lifestyle is crucial, but this book takes a step further by offering practical and actionable guidance. Recognizing that knowledge alone may not be enough for individuals to successfully adopt and maintain a low-carb approach, the book provides tangible strategies to bridge the gap between theory and practical application. Readers will discover comprehensive guidance on crafting balanced meal plans, navigating social situations, incorporating physical activity, and addressing emotional well-being. These actionable insights are designed to empower individuals, enabling them to seamlessly integrate a low-carb lifestyle into their daily routines.

The practical guidance in the book emphasizes the importance of crafting balanced meal plans. It goes beyond outlining the principles of a low-carb diet to provide concrete examples and strategies for creating meals that align with low-carb principles while being nutritionally rich and satisfying. This hands-on approach ensures that readers have the tools they need to implement dietary changes effectively and with a focus on overall well-being.

Social situations can pose challenges for individuals following specific dietary patterns, and this book acknowledges this reality while offering practical advice on navigating such scenarios. Whether it's dining out, attending social gatherings, or managing family meals, readers will find actionable strategies for making healthful choices without feeling restricted or isolated.

The significance of physical activity is emphasized, and the book provides guidance on seamlessly incorporating exercise into a low-carb lifestyle. By offering practical tips and suggestions, readers can discover enjoyable and sustainable ways to enhance their overall well-being through movement and activity.

Addressing emotional well-being is another aspect of the practical guidance provided. Recognizing the role of emotions in eating habits, the book offers strategies for fostering a positive relationship with food and managing stress without resorting to unhealthy dietary patterns.

Essentially, the practical guidance in the book extends beyond theory, providing readers with actionable steps to apply their knowledge in real-life situations. Covering aspects such as meal planning, social dynamics, physical activity, and emotional well-being, the book equips individuals with the tools needed to seamlessly integrate a low-carb lifestyle into their daily routines. This practical approach enhances the likelihood of successfully adopting and adhering to the principles of a low-carb diet over the long term.

Sustainability and Long-Term Success:

Recognizing the crucial nature of lasting lifestyle changes, this book places a strong emphasis on strategies designed for long-term success. Instead of concentrating solely on immediate outcomes, it delves into the intricacies of fostering enduring health improvements. The book provides valuable insights into overcoming challenges, setting realistic goals, and cultivating a mindset conducive to long-lasting well-being.

Understanding that achieving sustained lifestyle changes involves navigating various challenges, from the complexities of daily life to potential hurdles in adhering to a low-carb lifestyle, the book offers practical guidance on overcoming obstacles. By addressing common pitfalls and providing actionable solutions, it aims to empower readers with the resilience needed to successfully navigate challenges.

Establishing realistic goals is a fundamental element of the book's approach to long-term success. It goes beyond advocating for rapid or extreme changes, recognizing that gradual and sustainable progress is key. By providing insights into goal-setting strategies aligned with individual capabilities and preferences, the book encourages readers to adopt a realistic and achievable trajectory toward their health objectives.

A central tenet of the book's philosophy is its commitment to fostering a mindset conducive to lasting health improvements. This involves cultivating a positive and sustainable relationship with dietary choices, physical activity, and overall well-being. By offering tools for developing a mindset focused on long-term success, the book aims to instill habits that endure beyond short-lived trends or fads.

The ultimate goal, as emphasized by the book, extends beyond mere short-term weight loss. Instead, it centers on the establishment of enduring habits that contribute to overall well-being. By instilling a commitment to lasting health improvements, the book seeks to guide readers toward a lifestyle characterized by sustained vitality, improved health markers, and a holistic sense of well-being.

Holistic Approach:

Taking a holistic perspective is crucial, recognizing that health involves various aspects beyond dietary choices alone. This book embraces a comprehensive approach, delving into the intricate connections between nutrition, physical activity, mindfulness, and emotional well-being. Understanding the interplay of these elements, the book acts as a guide to help readers establish a well-rounded and holistic approach to health, surpassing the confines of a specific diet.

Health is a complex interweaving of multiple factors, and the book highlights the importance of considering the broader context in which dietary choices are situated. While nutrition is undeniably pivotal, the book offers in-depth insights into the principles of a low-carb lifestyle and goes further by integrating this nutritional guidance with other key components of well-being.

Physical activity is a central pillar in the holistic perspective promoted by the book. It stresses the significance of incorporating regular exercise into daily routines, not only for its physical benefits but also for its positive impact on mental health and overall vitality. By addressing the synergy between nutrition and physical activity, the book encourages readers to embrace a balanced and active lifestyle.

Mindfulness is another aspect explored in the book, recognizing the significance of conscious and intentional choices in nurturing a healthy relationship with food. By promoting mindful eating practices and highlighting the connection between the mind and body, the book assists readers in making considerate and informed decisions about their dietary habits.

Emotional well-being is also given thoughtful consideration. The book acknowledges the substantial impact emotions can have on dietary choices and overall health. Strategies for managing stress, addressing emotional triggers, and cultivating a positive mindset are intricately woven into the guidance provided by the book, offering readers a holistic approach to well-being.

By addressing these interrelated aspects of health, the book offers readers a guide for crafting a comprehensive and sustainable approach to their well-being. It underscores the understanding that optimal health isn't solely determined by adherence to a specific diet but emerges from the harmonious integration of nutrition, physical activity, mindfulness, and emotional well-being. In doing so, the book empowers individuals to embark on a holistic journey toward enduring health improvements and overall well-being.

Adaptability to Individual Needs:

Recognizing the inherent uniqueness of each individual, this book encourages readers to personalize the principles of Carbo-Conscious Living based on their specific needs and preferences. It highlights the importance of adaptability and flexibility, providing guidelines rather than imposing rigid rules. This approach empowers individuals to customize their low-carb lifestyle in a manner that aligns with their circumstances while staying true to the fundamental principles of this health-conscious approach.

In the realm of health and wellness, a one-size-fits-all approach is often impractical, given the diverse preferences, lifestyles, and health considerations of individuals. The book embraces this diversity and acknowledges that what works for one person may require adjustments for another. By promoting adaptability, it empowers readers to tailor the Carbo-Conscious Living principles to their unique situations, fostering a more sustainable and personalized approach to health.

The intentional emphasis on guidelines rather than strict rules allows for a more individualized application of the low-carb lifestyle. This approach recognizes that life is dynamic, with varying circumstances and preferences influencing dietary choices. By offering flexible guidelines, the book encourages readers to make informed decisions that suit their tastes, cultural backgrounds, and practical considerations while still adhering to the fundamental principles of a low-carb lifestyle.

In essence, the practical guidance provided in the book goes beyond theory, offering readers actionable steps to apply their knowledge in real-life situations. By addressing meal planning, social dynamics, physical activity, and emotional well-being, the book equips individuals with the tools needed to seamlessly integrate a low-carb lifestyle into their daily routines. This practical approach enhances the likelihood of successful adoption and long-term adherence to the principles of a low-carb diet.

Adaptability becomes a key theme, allowing individuals to seamlessly integrate the principles of Carbo-Conscious Living into their daily routines. Whether accommodating specific dietary preferences, managing unique health conditions, or navigating social and cultural contexts, the book empowers readers to make adjustments that suit their individual needs while staying aligned with the overarching philosophy of a low-carb lifestyle.

In essence, the book serves as a guide that respects and celebrates individual differences. It recognizes the diverse nature of personal preferences and health considerations, urging readers to view the principles of Carbo-Conscious Living as a flexible framework rather than a rigid set of rules. This approach not only fosters a sense of ownership over one's health journey but also promotes a sustainable and adaptable approach to embracing a low-carb lifestyle tailored to the uniqueness of each individual.

Inspiration and Motivation:

In essence, the practical guidance provided in the book goes beyond theory, offering readers actionable steps to apply their knowledge in real-life situations. By addressing meal planning, social dynamics, physical activity, and emotional well-being, the book equips individuals with the tools needed to seamlessly integrate a low-carb lifestyle into their daily routines. This practical approach enhances the likelihood of successful adoption and long-term adherence to the principles of a low-carb diet.

The primary aim is to serve as a source of inspiration and motivation for individuals embarking on their health journey. Utilizing success stories, practical examples, and a positive, encouraging tone, the intent is to instill confidence and enthusiasm in readers as they navigate the transformative path of Carbo-Conscious Living.

Success stories are powerful narratives that resonate with readers, offering tangible proof of the positive impact that embracing a low-carb lifestyle can have on individuals' health and well-being. By sharing these stories, the book aims to inspire readers, providing real-world examples of individuals who have successfully navigated the challenges and achieved notable health improvements through Carbo-Conscious Living.

Practical examples serve as relatable illustrations, demonstrating how the principles of Carbo-Conscious Living can be seamlessly integrated into everyday life. Through tangible scenarios and actionable tips, readers are guided on how to implement these principles in practical and achievable ways. This hands-on approach aims to empower individuals, making the transformative journey towards better health feel both accessible and realistic.

In essence, the practical guidance provided in the book goes beyond theory, offering readers actionable steps to apply their knowledge in real-life situations. By addressing meal planning, social dynamics, physical activity, and emotional well-being, the book equips individuals with the tools needed to seamlessly integrate a low-carb lifestyle into their daily routines. This practical approach enhances the likelihood of successful adoption and long-term adherence to the principles of a low-carb diet.

The tone adopted in the book is one of positivity and encouragement. Recognizing that embarking on a health journey, particularly one involving dietary changes, can be a challenging endeavor, the book seeks to create a supportive and uplifting atmosphere. The positive tone is intended to motivate readers, fostering a mindset of optimism and resilience as they navigate the various aspects of Carbo-Conscious Living.

The overarching goal is not only to provide information but to create an emotionally resonant and empowering experience for readers. By combining success stories, practical examples, and a positive tone, the book aspires to be a catalyst for motivation, inspiring individuals to take charge of their health and embrace Carbo-Conscious Living with confidence and enthusiasm.

Resource for Ongoing Support:

Recognizing that the pursuit of health is an ongoing and dynamic journey, the book positions itself as an indispensable resource for continued support. Its role extends beyond initial guidance, aiming to be a reliable companion throughout the entirety of readers' Carbo-Conscious Living experiences. To facilitate this ongoing support, the book equips individuals with tools for tracking progress, suggests adjustments as needed, and directs readers to additional resources, ensuring they have a comprehensive guide at every step of their health journey.

One key aspect of the book's ongoing support is the provision of tools for tracking progress. Recognizing the importance of measurable outcomes in sustaining motivation, the book offers practical methods for individuals to monitor their advancements in health and well-being. Whether it's tracking weight loss, changes in energy levels, or improvements in other health markers, these tools serve as tangible indicators of progress, reinforcing a sense of achievement and providing motivation for continued commitment.

In addition to tracking progress, the book offers valuable suggestions for adjustments. The journey to better health is not a straight path, and individuals may face challenges or need to modify their approach over time. By guiding potential adjustments and insights into common challenges, the book empowers readers to navigate obstacles effectively and make informed decisions about their Carbo-Conscious Living journey.

Moreover, the book directs readers to additional resources, recognizing that a comprehensive support system contributes to sustained success. Whether it's reputable websites, community forums, or other educational materials, the book serves as a gateway to a wealth of information that can enhance readers' understanding and offer additional support. This approach ensures that individuals have access to a broader network of resources that complement and strengthen the principles of Carbo-Conscious Living.

By providing ongoing support through tools for progress tracking, suggestions for adjustments, and access to additional resources, the book positions itself as a reliable guide for individuals dedicated to the journey of Carbo-Conscious Living. This commitment to continuous support reflects an understanding that health is a lifelong pursuit, and the book aims to be a dependable companion, offering guidance, encouragement, and resources for individuals at every stage of their ongoing health and wellness journey.

In essence, the purpose of this book is to be a comprehensive and empowering resource, directing individuals toward sustained health and well-being through the principles of Carbo-Conscious Living. Whether readers are new to the low-carb lifestyle or looking to refine their existing practices, the book is intended to be a trusted companion on their journey to a healthier, more vibrant life.

Understanding Low-Carb Diets: Navigating the Path to Health

In the realm of nutrition and dietary strategies, low-carb diets have garnered significant attention for their potential to contribute to various health benefits. A low-carb diet, as the name suggests, is characterized by a deliberate reduction in the consumption of carbohydrates, particularly those derived from refined sugars and starches. This approach to eating is rooted in the recognition that excessive carbohydrate intake, especially of the highly processed variety, can have significant health implications.

Defining Low-Carb Diets:

At its core, a low-carb diet revolves around moderating the consumption of foods rich in carbohydrates, which include sugars, grains, legumes, and starchy vegetables. While there's no universally agreed-upon definition for what qualifies as "low-carb," general guidelines typically involve a substantial decrease in daily carbohydrate intake compared to the prevalent Western diet where carbohydrates often make up the majority of daily calories.

The fundamental principle of a low-carb diet involves a deliberate and strategic reduction of carbohydrates, a primary macronutrient present in various food sources. Carbohydrates, found in sugars, grains, legumes, and specific vegetables, traditionally serve as a major energy source in diets. However, the low-carb approach challenges this norm by advocating for a decreased dependence on carbohydrates for energy.

The absence of a universally defined threshold for "low-carb" allows for flexibility in interpreting and applying the concept. Nonetheless, common guidelines recommend a significant cutback in daily carbohydrate intake compared to traditional dietary patterns. By doing so, individuals embracing a low-carb approach aim to shift their metabolic reliance from carbohydrates to alternative energy sources like fats and proteins.

In the typical Western diet, carbohydrates often make up the primary source of calories. The low-carb philosophy signifies a departure from this norm. By decreasing the percentage of daily calories obtained from carbohydrates, individuals commonly aim for metabolic advantages, such as enhanced weight management, better control of blood sugar levels, and overall metabolic health.

Types of Low-Carb Diets:

In the realm of low-carb diets, various versions exist, each with distinct principles and limitations tailored to specific health objectives. One widely recognized variant is the ketogenic diet, known for its extremely low-carb approach that triggers the body to enter a metabolic state called ketosis. During ketosis, the body primarily uses fat for energy, leading to weight loss and various metabolic advantages. Other notable variations include the Atkins Diet, which involves different phases of carbohydrate restriction, and the Paleo Diet, emphasizes whole, unprocessed foods like lean proteins and non-starchy vegetables.

The ketogenic diet is notable for its strict limitation of carbohydrates, typically restricting daily intake to a minimal amount. This prompts the production of ketones, molecules formed when fats break down, becoming the main energy source for the body. The ketogenic diet has gained popularity for its potential to aid weight loss, enhance blood sugar control, and improve mental clarity.

The Atkins Diet, another well-known low-carb variant, follows a phased approach to carbohydrate restriction. It starts with a more restrictive phase, significantly reducing carbohydrate intake, followed by a gradual reintroduction of carbs in subsequent phases. This tiered strategy allows individuals to adjust their carbohydrate intake based on progress and personal preferences, providing a flexible and adaptable approach to carb-conscious living.

The Paleo Diet, while not strictly categorized as a low-carb diet, often shares principles with low-carb approaches. Prioritizing whole, unprocessed foods, the Paleo Diet encourages the intake of lean proteins, fruits, vegetables, nuts, and seeds while discouraging grains, legumes, and processed foods. This dietary philosophy aims to mirror the eating patterns of our prehistoric ancestors, promoting a diet rich in nutrients and minimally processed foods.

These variations within the low-carb category showcase the diversity of dietary options, emphasizing that there isn't a one-size-fits-all approach. Individuals can select a low-carb variant that suits their preferences, health objectives, and lifestyle. Whether opting for the strict ketosis of the ketogenic diet, the phased approach of Atkins, or the whole-food emphasis of Paleo, these variations highlight the adaptability and personalization inherent in the low-carb philosophy.

How the Body Processes Carbohydrates:

To fully comprehend the reasoning behind low-carb diets, it's crucial to understand how carbohydrates affect the body. When consumed, carbohydrates undergo digestion, breaking down into glucose and causing an increase in blood sugar levels. In response to this elevation, the pancreas releases insulin, a hormone designed to aid the absorption of glucose into cells for energy use. Proponents of low-carb diets argue that reducing carbohydrate intake can be pivotal in maintaining stable blood sugar levels, potentially reducing the risk of insulin resistance and associated health issues.

The essential process of carbohydrate metabolism initiates with their digestion, leading to the breakdown into glucose. Glucose, serving as a primary energy source for the body, enters the bloodstream, causing a spike in blood sugar levels. This surge triggers the pancreas to release insulin, a hormone responsible for regulating glucose levels by facilitating its uptake into cells, where it can be utilized for energy production.

Supporters of low-carb diets assert that the regular consumption of high levels of carbohydrates, especially refined sugars and starches, can result in frequent spikes in blood sugar levels. Over time, the body may become less responsive to insulin, leading to a condition known as insulin resistance. This decreased sensitivity to insulin can contribute to elevated blood sugar levels and, ultimately, may give rise to health issues like type 2 diabetes and metabolic syndrome.

Low-carb diets advocate for a reduction in carbohydrate intake to minimize the frequency and intensity of blood sugar spikes. This approach places less strain on the pancreas to release significant amounts of insulin. The anticipated outcome is improved blood sugar control, which proponents argue can lower the risk of insulin resistance and its associated health complications.

In essence, the rationale behind low-carb diets lies in the understanding of how carbohydrates influence blood sugar levels and insulin response. Advocates propose that by moderating carbohydrate intake, individuals may potentially stabilize blood sugar levels, reduce the risk of insulin resistance, and address related health concerns. This perspective highlights the nuanced approach that low-carb diets take toward managing metabolic health and underscores the intricate interplay between diet, blood sugar regulation, and insulin sensitivity.

Benefits of a Low-Carb Lifestyle:

The decision to adopt a low-carb lifestyle is often motivated by a range of health benefits that extend beyond simple weight management. One significant factor is the positive impact on weight, as the decrease in carbohydrate intake is frequently associated with lower overall calorie consumption and subsequent fat loss. Additionally, low-carb diets have shown promise in improving markers related to cardiovascular health, such as reducing triglyceride levels and increasing high-density lipoprotein (HDL) cholesterol. For individuals dealing with conditions like diabetes, careful management of carbohydrate intake is crucial for achieving stability in blood sugar levels.

Weight management emerges as a compelling incentive for many individuals embracing a low-carb lifestyle. By moderating carbohydrate intake, individuals often witness a decrease in overall calorie consumption. This reduction, coupled with the body's transition to alternative energy sources, commonly results in fat loss. The controlled carbohydrate approach is acknowledged for its potential effectiveness in supporting weight loss endeavors, making it a popular choice among those aiming to manage their weight effectively.

Low-carb diets offer significant advantages for cardiovascular health, enhancing their attractiveness to many. Research indicates that these dietary patterns can contribute to a reduction in triglyceride levels, which are linked to heart health. Furthermore, these diets have demonstrated the ability to increase levels of HDL cholesterol, often known as the "good" cholesterol. These positive changes in lipid profiles suggest potential cardiovascular benefits, making low-carb lifestyles an appealing option for individuals seeking to enhance their heart health.

For those dealing with conditions such as diabetes, managing carbohydrate intake plays a crucial role in stabilizing blood sugar levels. Adopting a low-carb approach allows individuals to minimize the fluctuations in blood glucose associated with high carbohydrate consumption. This level of dietary control is particularly significant for individuals with diabetes, as it can assist in achieving better glycemic control and may reduce the need for insulin or other medications.

In conclusion, the decision to embrace a low-carb lifestyle is multifaceted and often originates from a desire to attain various health benefits. Beyond weight management, low-carb diets show promise in positively impacting cardiovascular health markers and play a critical role in stabilizing blood sugar levels, especially for those with conditions such as diabetes. This holistic approach to health underscores the versatility of low-carb lifestyles in addressing diverse health concerns and aligns with the broader trend of personalized and targeted dietary strategies for optimal well-being.

Considerations for a Balanced Approach:

Achieving a balanced low-carb diet goes beyond just limiting carbohydrate intake; it emphasizes the importance of choosing nutrient-dense, whole foods. This involves incorporating a variety of non-starchy vegetables, lean proteins, healthy fats, and, in certain cases, low-sugar fruits. The primary goal is not only to control carbohydrate consumption but, importantly, to ensure that the body receives essential nutrients crucial for overall health and well-being.

Non-starchy vegetables form the foundation of a balanced low-carb diet. Packed with vitamins, minerals, and dietary fiber, these vegetables offer a spectrum of nutrients essential for optimal health. Their Low-Carbohydrate content aligns with the principles of a low-carb lifestyle while guaranteeing a robust intake of vital micronutrients crucial for various physiological functions.

Lean proteins play a crucial role in a balanced low-carb diet, providing essential amino acids necessary for muscle maintenance, repair, and overall bodily function. Including proteins from sources like poultry, fish, lean meats, and plant-based options ensures a well-rounded nutrient profile while contributing to satiety, a key aspect of long-term adherence to a low-carb lifestyle.

Healthy fats are another essential component, acting as a valuable energy source and aiding in the absorption of fat-soluble vitamins. Avocado, olive oil, nuts, and seeds exemplify nutrient-dense sources of healthy fats that align with the principles of a balanced low-carb diet. By incorporating these fats, individuals can achieve a satisfying and sustainable dietary approach while optimizing their intake of essential nutrients.

In specific instances, low-sugar fruits are incorporated to provide natural sweetness and additional nutritional benefits to the diet. Berries, for instance, are abundant in antioxidants, vitamins, and fiber while containing relatively lower amounts of sugar compared to other fruits. This careful inclusion allows individuals to savor the flavors of fruit while maintaining a focus on moderating carbohydrate intake.

The ultimate goal of a balanced low-carb diet goes beyond simple carbohydrate restriction, aiming to ensure that the body receives a comprehensive spectrum of essential nutrients. Through the incorporation of nutrient-dense, whole foods, individuals can optimize their health while adhering to the principles of a low-carb lifestyle. This nuanced approach not only addresses carbohydrate moderation but also promotes a holistic and sustainable dietary pattern that supports overall well-being.

In conclusion, a low-carb diet is a strategic reduction in carbohydrate intake to achieve various health objectives. Whether the aim is weight management, improved blood sugar control, or enhanced overall well-being, individuals adopting a low-carb lifestyle follow a path that prioritizes mindful food choices and strives for a balanced, sustainable approach to nutrition.

Weight Management and Low-Carb Diets: A Strategic Alliance

One of the primary motivations for embracing a low-carb lifestyle is its efficacy in weight management. A well-structured low-carb diet offers individuals a strategic and science-backed approach to not only shedding excess pounds but also maintaining a healthy body weight. Understanding the complex relationship between low-carb diets and weight management is crucial for those seeking sustainable and long-term success in their health journey.

Caloric Restriction and Fat Utilization:

The foundational principle of weight management in a low-carb diet centers around caloric restriction. By intentionally limiting carbohydrate intake, individuals naturally reduce their overall caloric consumption. This reduction, combined with the body's adaptation to utilizing alternative fuel sources in the absence of carbohydrates, often leads to the utilization of stored fat for energy. This fundamental shift towards fat metabolism can significantly contribute to fat loss and, consequently, facilitate weight reduction.

Carbohydrates are a primary source of energy in the typical diet, and their restriction in a low-carb approach initiates a series of metabolic changes. The body, no longer primarily relying on carbohydrates for energy, seeks alternative fuel sources. In this situation, stored fat becomes a readily available reservoir, and the body begins breaking down fat into ketones, which serve as an alternative energy source.

The caloric restriction inherent in a low-carb diet plays a pivotal role in weight management. When individuals limit their carbohydrate intake, they naturally decrease the total number of calories consumed. This reduction creates a caloric deficit, a fundamental principle for weight loss, as the body starts utilizing stored fat to meet its energy needs.

The shift towards fat metabolism is particularly notable during a state of ketosis, a metabolic condition induced by low-carb diets. In ketosis, the body primarily relies on fat-derived ketones for energy, leading to increased fat oxidation. This heightened fat utilization contributes to the breakdown of stored fat deposits, resulting in weight loss over time.

It's crucial to recognize that the weight management benefits of a low-carb diet extend beyond mere caloric restriction. The metabolic adaptations, including the transition to fat metabolism, offer a unique advantage in targeting stored fat for energy, providing a more efficient pathway for weight reduction.

In summary, at the core of weight management in a low-carb diet is the principle of caloric restriction, achieved through the intentional reduction of carbohydrate intake. This reduction prompts the body to shift towards alternative fuel sources, predominantly utilizing stored fat for energy. The resulting metabolic changes, particularly during states of ketosis, contribute to increased fat oxidation and, consequently, weight loss. This multifaceted approach underscores the effectiveness of low-carb diets in addressing weight management through a combination of caloric control and metabolic adaptations.

Stabilizing Blood Sugar Levels:

Low-carb diets are carefully designed to counteract the spikes and crashes in blood sugar levels commonly associated with high-carbohydrate meals.

Stabilizing blood sugar is a crucial element of these diets, and its significance extends to weight management by regulating insulin secretion. Elevated insulin levels are often linked to increased fat storage, and by maintaining stable blood sugar, low-carb diets aim to create a more favorable environment for fat utilization, ultimately supporting weight loss.

The prevalent Western diet, characterized by high carbohydrate intake, frequently results in rapid increases in blood sugar levels after meals. This surge prompts the pancreas to release insulin, facilitating the absorption of glucose into cells. The subsequent decline in blood sugar levels can lead to feelings of fatigue and increased hunger, prompting the consumption of more carbohydrates and perpetuating a cycle of spikes and crashes.

Low-carb diets break the cycle by reducing carbohydrate intake, leading to slower and more controlled increases in blood sugar after meals. This measured response minimizes the necessity for sharp insulin spikes, fostering a more stable blood sugar environment. This stability is pivotal for weight management as it regulates the secretion of insulin, a hormone crucial for fat storage and metabolism.

Elevated insulin levels have been linked to increased fat storage in the body. When insulin is abundant, it instructs cells to take up glucose for energy and store excess glucose as fat. By moderating carbohydrate intake and stabilizing blood sugar levels, low-carb diets aim to decrease the need for excessive insulin secretion. This, in turn, establishes a more favorable metabolic environment, potentially encouraging the use of stored fat for energy and supporting weight loss.

The stabilization of blood sugar levels on a low-carb diet not only addresses immediate energy fluctuations but also contributes to a broader metabolic balance. By promoting steady blood sugar levels and minimizing the need for elevated insulin, low-carb diets strive to create an environment that encourages the body to utilize stored fat as an energy source. This comprehensive approach aligns with the overarching goal of weight management and emphasizes the intricate connection between dietary choices, blood sugar regulation, insulin sensitivity, and the body's utilization of stored fat.

Appetite Regulation and Satiety:

In a low-carb diet, where there is a higher emphasis on protein and healthy fats, composition plays a crucial role in managing appetite. The intentional inclusion of protein, found in sources like lean meats, poultry, fish, eggs, and plant-based alternatives, is well-known for its satisfying effect, helping individuals feel full for longer periods and reducing the likelihood of overeating. At the same time, the integration of healthy fats contributes to a sense of fullness, supporting individuals in adhering to portion control and making sustainable food choices.

Protein, considered an essential macronutrient, is abundant in various foods and is recognized for inducing a feeling of fullness, known as satiety. This effect results from the intricate process of protein digestion, triggering the release of hormones that signal to the brain that the body's nutritional needs are met. Consequently, those following a low-carb diet, which emphasizes protein-rich foods, are more likely to experience prolonged feelings of fullness, reducing the inclination to consume excess calories.

Healthy fats, a fundamental component of the low-carb diet, play a crucial role in controlling appetite. In contrast to simple carbohydrates, which can cause rapid spikes and crashes in blood sugar levels, fats offer a sustained and steady source of energy. This enduring energy release helps prevent sudden hunger pangs often associated with fluctuations in blood sugar. Additionally, fats take a longer time to digest, extending the feeling of fullness and aiding individuals in maintaining portion control during meals.

The interplay of protein and healthy fats in a low-carb diet creates a synergistic impact on appetite regulation. While protein induces an immediate feeling of fullness, healthy fats contribute to prolonged satiety, collectively working to reduce excessive food intake. This dual mechanism assists individuals in better managing their hunger levels, making it easier to follow portion control guidelines and adopt sustainable food choices in the long run.

In conclusion, the purposeful structure of a low-carb diet, featuring increased protein and healthy fat content, is strategically crafted to control appetite. By generating sensations of fullness and fostering sustained satiety, this dietary strategy assists individuals in effectively managing their hunger, lowering the chances of overeating, and enhancing the overall success and sustainability of the low-carb lifestyle.

Reduction in Water Weight:

When individuals start a low-carb diet, they often experience a reduction in water weight during the initial phase, and it's essential for those undertaking this dietary approach to comprehend this occurrence. Carbohydrates stored in the body contribute to water retention, and as carb intake diminishes, the body sheds excess water. While the initial drop in weight on the scale might be noticeable, individuals must realize that this doesn't signify long-term fat loss. Sustained weight management on a low-carb diet depends on the ongoing commitment to the principles of this lifestyle.

Carbohydrates in the body are stored as glycogen, and each gram of glycogen is linked to water. When individuals embark on a low-carb diet and reduce their carbohydrate intake, the body begins using glycogen stores for energy. As glycogen is used up, the associated water is released, resulting in a rapid loss of water weight.

The decrease in water weight is often the first visible change when starting a low-carb diet. While this initial drop on the scale can be encouraging, individuals must understand that this is a temporary and anticipated phenomenon. The loss of water weight doesn't translate to long-term fat loss but signifies the depletion of stored carbohydrates and the associated water. For sustainable weight management on a low-carb diet, individuals must grasp this process and remain committed to the principles of the lifestyle.

For individuals aiming for lasting weight management and fat loss on a low-carb diet, it's crucial to consistently follow the principles of this lifestyle. This entails maintaining a well-calibrated balance of macronutrients, ensuring sufficient protein and healthy fats while moderating carbohydrate intake. The key to achieving and sustaining a healthy weight over time lies in the steadfast adherence to these dietary choices, coupled with a mindful approach to overall caloric intake.

The decrease in water weight observed in the initial phase of a low-carb diet emphasizes the importance of recognizing that the scale isn't the sole measure of progress. While the initial decline may encourage, the enduring impact on long-term health and body composition stems from unwavering dedication to the principles of the low-carb lifestyle. Through this commitment, individuals can attain not only a temporary reduction in water weight but also a lasting and significant transformation in their overall health and well-being.

Improved Metabolic Health:

The benefits of weight management on a low-carb diet go beyond simple changes in numbers on the scale, extending to a profound impact on metabolic health. Many individuals who adopt a low-carb lifestyle witness significant improvements in key health markers, including triglyceride levels, blood pressure, and insulin sensitivity. These positive changes not only enhance overall health but also create an environment conducive to sustained and long-term weight management.

Triglyceride levels, a crucial component of lipid profiles, often undergo positive transformations in response to a low-carb diet. Elevated triglycerides are associated with an increased risk of cardiovascular issues. However, individuals adhering to a low-carb approach commonly experience a reduction in triglyceride levels, promoting cardiovascular health and mitigating potential risks.

Blood pressure, another vital metric linked to cardiovascular well-being, frequently demonstrates favorable changes on a low-carb diet. The reduction in carbohydrate intake contributes to improved blood pressure control, thereby alleviating strain on the cardiovascular system. These enhancements in blood pressure have broader implications for heart health and contribute to an overall reduction in cardiovascular risk.

Insulin sensitivity, a crucial aspect of metabolic health, experiences positive effects with the adoption of a low-carb lifestyle. Insulin, a hormone responsible for regulating blood sugar levels, becomes more efficient in managing glucose, leading to enhanced sensitivity. Improved insulin sensitivity is associated with a reduced risk of type 2 diabetes and metabolic syndrome, both of which are linked to long-term health complications.

The alterations in triglyceride levels, blood pressure, and insulin sensitivity signify not only enhancements in metabolic health but also create a conducive environment for sustained weight management. The intricate interplay between metabolic markers and weight management goes beyond mere aesthetics, extending to broader aspects of overall well-being.

The holistic nature of a low-carb diet addresses not only weight but also various facets of metabolic health. It illuminates the intricate connections between dietary choices, metabolic markers, and overall well-being. By fostering positive changes in triglyceride levels, blood pressure, and insulin sensitivity, individuals embracing a low-carb lifestyle position themselves for not only successful weight management but also comprehensive improvement in their metabolic health and long-term vitality.

Long-Term Sustainability:

The effectiveness of weight management on a low-carb diet is closely linked to the sustainability inherent in its approach. Unlike fad diets that pledge rapid results but often prove difficult to maintain over the long term, the low-carb lifestyle advocates for a balanced and sustainable approach to nutrition. Prioritizing the consumption of whole, nutrient-dense foods and accommodating individual dietary preferences, low-carb diets are crafted to seamlessly integrate into one's lifestyle for sustained, long-term success.

Fad diets often entice individuals with promises of quick and dramatic weight loss. However, the restrictive nature of many fad diets, combined with their tendency to exclude entire food groups or rely on overly complicated meal plans, frequently leads to challenges in adherence. Such diets are typically characterized by a short-term focus, with the initial enthusiasm diminishing over time as individuals find them challenging to sustain.

In contrast, the low-carb lifestyle embraces a holistic and realistic perspective on nutrition. Instead of imposing rigid rules, it encourages individuals to make mindful and balanced choices, emphasizing the incorporation of whole, nutrient-dense foods. This flexibility fosters a more personalized and adaptable approach, accommodating individual preferences and variations in lifestyle.

The sustainability of a low-carb diet is grounded in its focus on whole foods. By giving priority to nutrient-dense sources of carbohydrates, proteins, and fats, individuals can obtain essential nutrients while moderating their carbohydrate intake. This not only supports weight management but also contributes to overall well-being and health.

Moreover, the low-carb lifestyle acknowledges and respects individual dietary preferences, making it more likely for individuals to adhere to the principles of the diet over the long term. Whether someone opts for a plant-based approach, includes dairy in their diet, or follows specific cultural or culinary preferences, the low-carb framework can be adapted to meet diverse needs.

Essentially, the sustainability of weight management on a low-carb diet stems from its realistic and adaptable nature. By endorsing a balanced approach to nutrition, incorporating whole, nutrient-dense foods, and accommodating individual preferences, the low-carb lifestyle is crafted to be a viable and enduring choice. This emphasis on long-term sustainability sets it apart from transient fad diets, positioning it as a practical and effective strategy for those seeking not only short-term weight loss but also lasting health and well-being.

Weight management on a low-carb diet involves a dynamic interplay of caloric restriction, metabolic adaptations, and mindful food choices. By comprehending the mechanisms at play and adopting a holistic approach to health, individuals can leverage the benefits of a low-carb lifestyle for effective and sustainable weight management.

Blood Sugar Control and the Low-Carb Lifestyle: A Balancing Act for Health

One of the compelling advantages of adopting a low-carb lifestyle is its impact on blood sugar control. For individuals grappling with conditions like diabetes or seeking to prevent insulin resistance, a low-carb diet offers a strategic and science-backed approach to managing blood sugar levels. Understanding the intricate relationship between carbohydrate intake and blood sugar regulation is pivotal in appreciating the benefits of the low-carb lifestyle.

Stabilizing Blood Glucose Levels:

At the core of the low-carb lifestyle is the purposeful decrease in carbohydrate intake, a critical component in stabilizing blood glucose levels. By moderating the consumption of sugars and starches, individuals can effectively minimize the swift spikes in blood glucose that often follow meals rich in carbohydrates. This deliberate reduction in post-meal blood sugar fluctuations holds significant benefits, particularly for individuals with diabetes, assisting them in maintaining more stable and healthier blood sugar levels throughout the day.

Carbohydrates serve as a primary source of glucose, the primary form of sugar in the bloodstream. Upon consumption, carbohydrates are broken down into glucose, leading to an elevation in blood sugar levels. For individuals with diabetes, the body's ability to regulate blood sugar is compromised, necessitating careful management of carbohydrate intake to avoid abrupt spikes in glucose levels.

The deliberate reduction of carbohydrates in the low-carb lifestyle empowers individuals to regulate the impact of their dietary choices on blood glucose. Steering clear of excessive sugars and starches allows for a more gradual and controlled release of glucose into the bloodstream. This measured response reduces the body's reliance on producing substantial amounts of insulin to facilitate glucose uptake, fostering steadier and healthier blood sugar levels.

This nuanced approach to moderating carbohydrate intake is particularly advantageous for individuals with diabetes, where maintaining stable blood glucose levels is of paramount importance. Fluctuations in blood sugar can contribute to various health issues, including heightened insulin resistance, fatigue, and complications associated with poorly managed diabetes. Embracing a low-carb lifestyle enables individuals with diabetes to actively manage their carbohydrate intake, promoting more stable blood sugar levels and mitigating the risk of these complications.

Insulin Sensitivity and Reduction of Insulin Resistance:

Insulin, a pivotal hormone produced by the pancreas, plays a crucial role in regulating blood sugar levels. Prolonged exposure to elevated levels of carbohydrates can lead to a condition known as insulin resistance, where cells become less responsive to insulin signals. A low-carb diet is strategically designed to address and enhance insulin sensitivity, promoting the body's ability to utilize insulin more effectively. This improvement in sensitivity facilitates the efficient transport of glucose into cells for energy, ultimately contributing to better blood sugar control.

Insulin functions as a key mediator in the body's glucose metabolism. When carbohydrates are consumed, the pancreas releases insulin to facilitate the absorption and utilization of glucose by cells. However, continuous exposure to high levels of carbohydrates, especially refined sugars and starches, can induce a state of insulin resistance. In this condition, cells no longer respond efficiently to insulin signals, resulting in elevated blood sugar levels and an increased demand for insulin production.

A fundamental objective of a low-carb diet is to improve insulin sensitivity. By reducing the consumption of carbohydrates, especially those that cause rapid spikes in blood sugar, the body's reliance on insulin is moderated. This reduction in carbohydrate intake helps break the cycle of continuous high insulin levels, allowing cells to regain their responsiveness to insulin signals.

Enhanced insulin sensitivity yields several positive effects on blood sugar management. When cells respond more effectively to insulin, the transport of glucose into cells becomes more efficient. This means that the body can utilize glucose for energy without requiring excessive amounts of insulin. The improved ability of cells to take up glucose contributes to better blood sugar control and a reduced risk of complications associated with insulin resistance, such as type 2 diabetes.

In summary, a low-carb diet aims to address insulin resistance by improving insulin sensitivity. By strategically moderating carbohydrate intake, the diet allows the body to utilize insulin more efficiently, facilitating the optimal transport of glucose into cells for energy. This improvement in insulin sensitivity contributes to better blood sugar control, aligning with the overall goal of promoting metabolic health and reducing the risk of complications associated with insulin resistance.

Impact on Hemoglobin A1c Levels:

Hemoglobin A1c, a crucial marker used to assess average blood sugar levels over several months, is particularly important for individuals dealing with diabetes. Studies suggest that adherence to a low-carb diet can result in significant improvements in Hemoglobin A1c levels, indicating enhanced long-term blood sugar control. This reduction in average blood sugar levels plays a crucial role in reducing the risk of complications associated with diabetes.

Hemoglobin A1c, commonly abbreviated as HbA1c, offers a comprehensive representation of blood sugar control over an extended period. It measures the percentage of hemoglobin that has become glycated or bound to glucose in the bloodstream. Since red blood cells have a lifespan of approximately three months, HbA1c levels reflect the average blood sugar concentration during this timeframe. For individuals managing diabetes, maintaining optimal HbA1c levels is a key objective in preventing complications linked to prolonged exposure to elevated blood sugar.

Numerous studies have delved into the effects of a low-carb diet on Hemoglobin A1c levels, consistently revealing positive outcomes. Embracing a low-carb lifestyle has been linked to reductions in HbA1c levels, signaling improved long-term blood sugar control. This enhancement holds particular significance for individuals with diabetes, as elevated HbA1c levels are associated with an increased risk of complications, including cardiovascular issues, kidney problems, and nerve damage.

The impact of a low-carb diet on Hemoglobin A1c levels lies in its ability to regulate blood sugar. By moderating carbohydrate intake, the diet helps prevent sudden spikes in blood sugar, fostering a more stable and controlled glucose environment. Consequently, this contributes to lower average blood sugar levels over time, as evidenced by improved HbA1c measurements.

The decrease in Hemoglobin A1c levels achieved through a low-carb diet highlights the potential efficacy of this dietary approach in managing diabetes effectively. Beyond addressing day-to-day blood sugar fluctuations, the low-carb lifestyle takes a long-term perspective on diabetes management, assisting individuals in achieving and sustaining optimal HbA1c levels. This not only signifies enhanced blood sugar control but also plays a crucial role in diminishing the risk of diabetes-related complications, underscoring the pivotal role of dietary choices in the overall well-being of individuals managing diabetes.

Managing Hypoglycemia:

While low-carb diets excel in stabilizing blood sugar levels, individuals on specific medications or insulin therapy must be mindful of the potential risk of hypoglycemia, which is low blood sugar. To navigate this, close monitoring, adjustments to medication under medical supervision, and strategic meal planning become essential precautions to prevent episodes of hypoglycemia while embracing a low-carb lifestyle.

Low-carb diets inherently focus on moderating carbohydrate intake to enhance blood sugar control, offering significant benefits for many, especially those with conditions like diabetes. However, individuals relying on certain medications or insulin therapy to regulate their blood sugar levels may encounter an elevated risk of hypoglycemia when transitioning to a low-carb lifestyle.

Hypoglycemia occurs when blood sugar levels drop below normal, resulting in symptoms like dizziness, confusion, sweating, and, in severe cases, loss of consciousness. Individuals using medications or insulin to lower blood sugar face an increased risk of hypoglycemia when adopting a low-carb diet, as there are fewer carbohydrates available to raise blood sugar levels.

For those on medications or insulin therapy, close collaboration with healthcare professionals during the transition to a low-carb lifestyle is essential. This medical supervision ensures careful monitoring of blood sugar levels and necessary adjustments to medications, minimizing the risk of hypoglycemia while benefiting from improved blood sugar control.

Strategic meal planning plays a crucial role in managing hypoglycemia on a low-carb diet. Thoughtful consideration of meal timing and composition, including nutrient-dense, low-carbohydrate options, helps maintain stable blood sugar levels. The balance of protein, fats, and complex carbohydrates becomes instrumental in preventing sharp drops in blood sugar while providing sustained energy.

Individuals must be educated about recognizing the signs and symptoms of hypoglycemia and empowered to take appropriate action, such as consuming a small amount of glucose-containing food or beverage if needed. Regular self-monitoring of blood sugar levels is also recommended to track responses to dietary changes and medication adjustments.

In summary, while low-carb diets offer substantial benefits in stabilizing blood sugar levels, a cautious and collaborative approach is necessary for individuals on certain medications or insulin therapy. Through close collaboration with healthcare professionals, engaging in strategic meal planning, and maintaining vigilant monitoring, individuals can safely and effectively navigate a low-carb lifestyle, minimizing the risk of hypoglycemia and optimizing their overall health.

Individualized Approach to Carbohydrate Tolerance:

The low-carb lifestyle acknowledges and emphasizes the significance of individualized approaches to carbohydrate tolerance. Recognizing that people vary in their responses to dietary changes, the low-carb philosophy encourages a personalized approach where individuals can tailor their carbohydrate intake to align with their unique needs. While some individuals may thrive on very low-carb diets, others may find that a more moderate or flexible approach better suits their requirements. Understanding one's own carbohydrate tolerance and making adjustments based on personal responses are crucial aspects of blood sugar management within the low-carb framework.

Carbohydrate tolerance refers to an individual's capacity to metabolize and manage carbohydrates without experiencing adverse effects on blood sugar levels. It takes into consideration factors such as insulin sensitivity, metabolic rate, activity levels, and overall health. The low-carb lifestyle recognizes that there is no one-size-fits-all approach when it comes to carbohydrate intake, and what works optimally for one person may differ for another.

Some individuals may find that they thrive on very low-carb diets, which typically involve a significant reduction in daily carbohydrate intake. These individuals may experience improved blood sugar control, weight management, and other health benefits. On the other hand, some people may prefer or require a more moderate or flexible approach that allows for a slightly higher intake of carbohydrates, often sourced from nutrient-dense sources like vegetables, fruits, and whole grains.

The key to successfully navigating an individualized approach to carbohydrate tolerance lies in self-awareness and attentiveness to one's body's responses. It involves paying close attention to how different levels of carbohydrate intake impact energy levels, blood sugar readings, and overall well-being. Regular monitoring, along with adjustments based on personal responses, allows individuals to fine-tune their dietary choices to align with their specific needs and goals.

Education plays a crucial role in empowering individuals to understand their carbohydrate tolerance. By providing information on the principles of the low-carb lifestyle, the potential benefits of different carbohydrate levels, and the importance of self-monitoring, individuals can make informed decisions about their dietary choices.

In summary, the low-carb lifestyle underscores the importance of recognizing and embracing individualized approaches to carbohydrate tolerance. This flexible philosophy allows individuals to tailor their dietary choices to suit their unique needs, promoting better blood sugar management and overall health. Understanding one's carbohydrate tolerance and making adjustments based on personal responses foster a dynamic and personalized approach within the low-carb framework, supporting individuals in achieving their health and wellness goals.

Collaborative Approach with Healthcare Providers:

In the context of managing diabetes or other blood sugar-related conditions, a collaborative approach with healthcare providers is imperative when adopting a low-carb lifestyle. Close collaboration involves ongoing communication, monitoring of blood sugar levels, adjusting medications as needed, and seeking professional guidance. This collaborative effort ensures that the low-carb lifestyle is tailored to individual health needs and aligned with overall wellness goals.

Individuals managing diabetes or other conditions that affect blood sugar levels often require specialized care and support. Collaborating with healthcare providers, including physicians, registered dietitians, and diabetes educators, is crucial for ensuring that the low-carb approach is integrated safely and effectively into an individual's overall healthcare plan.

One key aspect of collaboration is regular monitoring of blood sugar levels. Healthcare providers can guide individuals on how to accurately measure and interpret their blood glucose readings. This ongoing monitoring helps assess the impact of the low-carb lifestyle on blood sugar control, allowing for timely adjustments to dietary choices, medications, or insulin regimens.

Adjusting medications, particularly those related to blood sugar management, is another critical element of the collaborative approach. As dietary changes can influence the need for certain medications, healthcare providers play a pivotal role in assessing and modifying medication regimens to align with the low-carb lifestyle. This ensures that individuals maintain optimal blood sugar control while minimizing the risk of hypoglycemia or other complications.

Professional guidance is essential for individuals navigating the complexities of blood sugar management within the low-carb framework. Healthcare providers can offer personalized recommendations based on an individual's medical history, current health status, and specific health goals. This guidance may include advice on the type and amount of carbohydrates to consume, meal planning strategies, and considerations for physical activity.

The collaborative approach extends beyond the initial adoption of the low-carb lifestyle. Regular follow-up appointments and ongoing communication with healthcare providers enable individuals to address any challenges, receive additional support, and make necessary adjustments to their dietary and lifestyle choices. This continuous dialogue ensures that the low-carb approach evolves in tandem with an individual's health needs and wellness objectives.

In conclusion, the low-carb lifestyle presents a powerful strategy for blood sugar control, offering individuals a means to stabilize glucose levels, improve insulin sensitivity, and manage diabetes more effectively. By adopting a mindful and intentional approach to carbohydrate intake, individuals can navigate their health journey to achieve and sustain optimal blood sugar control.

Elevated Energy Levels on a Low-Carb Diet: Unlocking Vitality through Nutritional Precision

One of the notable and often celebrated outcomes of adopting a low-carb lifestyle is the profound impact it can have on energy levels. Contrary to the misconception that reduced carbohydrate intake leads to fatigue, a well-structured low-carb diet strategically harnesses alternative energy sources, resulting in sustained and heightened vitality. Understanding how this dietary approach influences energy metabolism is essential for those seeking to optimize their daily performance and well-being.

Steady Blood Sugar Levels:

Achieving and maintaining steady blood sugar levels is a fundamental aspect of the low-carb lifestyle, crucial for sustaining energy throughout the day. This dietary approach is intentionally designed to minimize the consumption of rapidly digestible carbohydrates that can lead to spikes and crashes in blood glucose levels. Instead, the low-carb lifestyle encourages the consumption of nutrient-dense, slow-digesting foods, facilitating a steady and sustained release of glucose into the bloodstream. This steadiness in blood sugar levels contributes to a consistent and reliable energy supply.

Rapid fluctuations in blood sugar levels, often associated with the consumption of high-glycemic carbohydrates, can lead to energy peaks and subsequent crashes. The low-carb lifestyle strategically addresses this issue by advocating for a reduction in the intake of rapidly digestible carbohydrates, such as sugars and refined starches. By limiting these sources of quick energy, the diet helps prevent the sharp spikes in blood glucose that can result in feelings of fatigue, irritability, and cravings.

Instead of focusing on rapidly digestible carbohydrates, the low-carb lifestyle emphasizes nutrient-dense, slow-digesting foods that provide a sustained release of glucose into the bloodstream. These may include non-starchy vegetables, lean proteins, healthy fats, and, in some cases, moderate amounts of whole grains. Consuming carbohydrates in a form that takes longer to break down allows for a more gradual and controlled release of glucose, promoting a stable blood sugar environment.

The steadiness in blood sugar levels achieved through the low-carb lifestyle has significant implications for energy levels. A consistent and reliable supply of glucose supports sustained energy throughout the day, reducing the likelihood of energy dips and enhancing overall vitality. Individuals following a low-carb diet often report improved mental clarity, enhanced focus, and a more balanced mood due to the stable blood sugar levels facilitated by their dietary choices.

Additionally, the advantages of maintaining consistent blood sugar levels extend beyond immediate energy considerations. This approach is in harmony with the principles of blood sugar management, aiding individuals in reducing the risk of insulin resistance, effectively managing weight, and promoting overall metabolic health.

To sum up, the low-carb lifestyle places a priority on sustaining steady blood sugar levels as a crucial element of enduring energy. By minimizing rapidly digestible carbohydrates and emphasizing nutrient-dense, slow-digesting foods, this dietary approach ensures a reliable release of glucose into the bloodstream. This steadiness contributes to a consistent and lasting energy supply, fostering improved overall well-being and aligning with the principles of blood sugar management within the low-carb framework.

Transition to Fat Metabolism:

A fundamental aspect of the low-carb lifestyle revolves around orchestrating a metabolic shift within the body, transitioning from predominantly relying on carbohydrates for energy to tapping into stored fat. This metabolic transformation, commonly known as ketosis, occurs when intentional reductions in carbohydrate intake prompt the body to initiate the breakdown of fat for fuel. Consequently, ketones emerge as byproducts of fat metabolism, serving as an alternative energy source for both the brain and body. This shift to fat metabolism establishes a sustained and efficient energy source, representing a foundational principle of the low-carb lifestyle.

Ketosis is a metabolic state wherein the body starts producing and utilizing ketones as a primary energy source. This transition unfolds when carbohydrate intake is restricted, leading the body to deplete its glycogen stores—stored forms of glucose. In the absence of readily available glucose from carbohydrates, the body redirects its focus to breaking down stored fat into fatty acids and glycerol.

The breakdown of fats produces ketones, small molecules capable of crossing the blood-brain barrier and acting as an alternative fuel for both the brain and other tissues in the body. This shift to fat metabolism establishes a sustained and efficient energy source, in contrast to the fluctuations associated with the conventional reliance on carbohydrates.

One notable benefit of transitioning to fat metabolism through ketosis is the utilization of stored fat for fuel, leading to weight loss and changes in body composition. As the body taps into its fat reserves, individuals often experience a reduction in body fat, contributing to overall weight management.

Furthermore, the sustained energy derived from fat metabolism promotes improved endurance and stamina. While carbohydrates can offer quick bursts of energy, they are frequently followed by subsequent crashes. In contrast, the steady release of energy from the breakdown of fats in ketosis supports endurance, enabling individuals to maintain energy levels over extended periods.

It's crucial to understand that entering and sustaining ketosis requires a conscious reduction in carbohydrate intake, typically below the levels found in a traditional Western diet. This adjustment may entail a period during which the body adapts to the metabolic shift. Individuals adhering to a low-carb lifestyle often monitor their macronutrient intake, specifically moderating carbohydrates while ensuring sufficient consumption of proteins and healthy fats.

In summary, the shift to fat metabolism, facilitated by the low-carb lifestyle and characterized by ketosis, is a core principle of this dietary approach. This metabolic transition from reliance on carbohydrates to utilizing stored fat provides a consistent and efficient energy source through the production of ketones. Beyond its impact on weight management, the transition to fat metabolism contributes to enhanced endurance and stamina, making it a pivotal aspect of the metabolic adjustments associated with the low-carb lifestyle.

Enhanced Mitochondrial Function:

Mitochondria, recognized as the powerhouse of cells, play a crucial role in energy production within the human body. The low-carb lifestyle has been linked to significant enhancements in mitochondrial function, leading to improved cellular energy production. As the body adjusts to utilizing fats for energy, there is an increase in mitochondrial efficiency, ultimately boosting the overall capacity to generate adenosine triphosphate (ATP), which serves as the primary energy currency for cells.

Mitochondria, specialized cellular organelles, are responsible for ATP production through oxidative phosphorylation. ATP is vital for fueling various cellular functions, muscle contractions, and overall metabolic activities.

The low-carb lifestyle triggers a metabolic shift where the body prioritizes the use of fats, both from the diet and stored sources, for energy production. This shift is associated with enhancements in mitochondrial function. Mitochondria adapt to the increased reliance on fatty acids by improving their efficiency in generating ATP through oxidative phosphorylation.

Maintaining optimal cellular function and overall energy balance relies on the critical factor of mitochondrial efficiency. As mitochondrial ATP production becomes more efficient, cells can better meet their energy demands. This is particularly significant for tissues with elevated energy requirements, including muscles and organs involved in diverse metabolic processes.

The low-carb lifestyle, characterized by the adaptation to using fats for energy, triggers a process known as mitochondrial biogenesis. This process involves the formation of new mitochondria and the enhancement of existing ones. Through this adaptive response, the body maximizes its ability to produce ATP, fostering improved energy efficiency and resilience.

Elevated mitochondrial function extends beyond immediate energy production, impacting metabolic health, endurance, and overall well-being. Studies suggest that optimizing mitochondrial function might have implications for mitigating aging effects, promoting longevity, and enhancing cellular resilience against various stressors.

To summarize, the low-carb lifestyle, through its promotion of a metabolic shift towards utilizing fats for energy, has been linked to improvements in mitochondrial function. The heightened efficiency of ATP production within mitochondria contributes to enhanced cellular energy production and overall metabolic health. This facet of the low-carb lifestyle highlights its potential influence on optimizing cellular function, fostering resilience, and supporting the body's energy-producing capabilities by improving mitochondrial efficiency.

Reduction in Energy-Sapping Foods:

The low-carb lifestyle encourages a purposeful reduction or elimination of foods that can drain energy, such as processed items, refined sugars, and simple carbohydrates. These types of foods may cause fluctuations in energy levels. By focusing on the consumption of whole, nutrient-dense foods, individuals adhering to the low-carb lifestyle are less likely to experience the energy-draining effects associated with processed and sugary snacks. This dietary shift promotes sustained energy levels and reduces the necessity for frequent refueling.

Processed foods, often rich in added sugars and refined carbohydrates, can lead to quick spikes and subsequent crashes in blood sugar levels. These fluctuations contribute to feelings of fatigue, irritability, and a need for frequent snacking to maintain energy levels. The low-carb lifestyle addresses this issue strategically by encouraging individuals to limit or eliminate such energy-draining foods.

Refined sugars and simple carbohydrates, commonly found in processed snacks and sugary beverages, offer a quick but short-lived burst of energy, followed by a rapid decline. This rollercoaster effect on blood sugar levels can leave individuals feeling drained and in need of a quick energy boost. The low-carb lifestyle addresses this by reducing the intake of these types of carbohydrates, helping to stabilize blood sugar levels and resulting in more consistent and sustained energy throughout the day.

The foundation of the low-carb diet is built upon whole, nutrient-dense foods, including vegetables, fruits, lean proteins, and healthy fats. These foods are packed with essential nutrients, fiber, and slow-digesting carbohydrates. Unlike their processed counterparts, they contribute to a gradual release of glucose into the bloodstream, providing a sustained and reliable source of energy.

The emphasis on nutrient-dense choices aligns with the principle of nourishing the body with foods that support overall health and well-being. Nutrient-dense foods not only contribute to sustained energy levels but also offer a wealth of vitamins, minerals, and antioxidants that are beneficial for various bodily functions.

In addition to promoting sustained energy, reducing energy-sapping foods aligns with other health benefits linked to the low-carb lifestyle, such as weight management, improved metabolic health, and enhanced cognitive function. This approach guides individuals in making food choices that contribute to their overall vitality and diminishes the reliance on frequent snacks to maintain energy levels.

To summarize, the low-carb lifestyle advocates for a decrease in energy-sapping foods, emphasizing whole, nutrient-dense choices over processed and sugary snacks. By avoiding the rapid fluctuations in blood sugar levels associated with processed carbohydrates, individuals can experience more sustained energy throughout the day. This dietary approach not only supports energy levels but also aligns with broader health goals, underscoring the importance of nourishing the body with foods that contribute to overall well-being.

Improved Insulin Sensitivity:

Improved insulin sensitivity is a key benefit associated with the low-carb lifestyle, addressing concerns related to insulin resistance often associated with high-carbohydrate diets. Insulin resistance can contribute to feelings of fatigue and sluggishness. The low-carb lifestyle, by promoting insulin sensitivity, ensures that glucose is efficiently transported into cells for energy, preventing the energy-depleting effects of insulin resistance and supporting sustained vitality.

Insulin is a hormone produced by the pancreas that plays a crucial role in regulating blood sugar levels. Its primary function is to facilitate the uptake of glucose into cells, where it can be utilized for energy. However, when individuals consistently consume high amounts of carbohydrates, especially refined sugars, and starches, the body may become less responsive to insulin's signals. This phenomenon is known as insulin resistance.

Insulin resistance can result in elevated blood sugar levels as cells become less efficient at absorbing glucose. This can lead to increased insulin production in an attempt to compensate for the resistance, creating a cycle that may contribute to fatigue and a lack of vitality. The low-carb lifestyle addresses this by promoting improved insulin sensitivity.

By moderating carbohydrate intake and focusing on nutrient-dense, whole foods, the low-carb lifestyle helps prevent excessive fluctuations in blood sugar levels. This, in turn, supports the body in maintaining or improving its insulin sensitivity. When insulin sensitivity is enhanced, cells efficiently respond to insulin's signals, allowing for the effective transport of glucose into cells for energy production.

The promotion of insulin sensitivity is particularly significant for individuals seeking sustained vitality. When glucose is efficiently utilized for energy, individuals are less likely to experience the energy crashes associated with insulin resistance. Instead, they can enjoy a more consistent and sustained release of energy, contributing to improved overall well-being.

Additionally, improved insulin sensitivity aligns with broader health benefits, including better weight management and reduced risk of metabolic disorders. By preventing the negative effects of insulin resistance, the low-carb lifestyle supports not only immediate energy levels but also long-term health and vitality.

In summary, the low-carb lifestyle plays a crucial role in promoting improved insulin sensitivity. By moderating carbohydrate intake and emphasizing nutrient-dense foods, this dietary approach ensures efficient glucose transport into cells for energy production. The result is a reduction in the energy-depleting effects of insulin resistance, supporting individuals in experiencing sustained vitality and contributing to their overall health and well-being.

Cognitive Clarity

and Mental Energy:

Cognitive clarity and mental energy are notable benefits associated with a low-carb diet, demonstrating the impact of dietary choices on brain function. The stability of blood sugar levels and the brain's utilization of ketones for energy contribute to enhanced mental clarity, focus, and sustained cognitive function. Individuals following a low-carb diet often report improved productivity and alertness throughout the day.

The brain relies heavily on a stable and consistent supply of energy to function optimally. In a typical Western diet characterized by high carbohydrate intake, fluctuations in blood sugar levels can occur, leading to periods of mental fog, irritability, and difficulty concentrating. The low-carb lifestyle strategically addresses this issue by promoting stable blood sugar levels and minimizing the peaks and crashes associated with high-carbohydrate meals.

When carbohydrate intake is reduced, the body enters a state of ketosis, wherein it begins to produce and utilize ketones as an alternative energy source for the brain. Ketones are molecules produced during the breakdown of fats, and they can efficiently cross the blood-brain barrier to provide a consistent supply of energy to the brain. This metabolic adaptation is believed to contribute to the cognitive benefits observed in individuals following a low-carb diet.

Stable blood sugar levels and the reliance on ketones for brain energy contribute to enhanced mental clarity. Individuals often report improved focus, sharper cognitive function, and a sustained ability to concentrate on tasks. The absence of the energy crashes associated with fluctuating blood sugar levels allows for a more consistent and reliable mental state throughout the day.

Moreover, some research suggests that a low-carb diet may have neuro-protective effects and could potentially reduce the risk of neurodegenerative conditions. By providing a stable and efficient source of energy to the brain, the low-carb lifestyle supports cognitive health and may contribute to long-term brain function.

Individuals following a low-carb diet often describe an improvement in productivity and alertness. The cognitive benefits extend beyond immediate mental clarity, influencing overall mental well-being and daily performance. Many report feeling more mentally energized, leading to a greater capacity to tackle tasks, make decisions, and sustain mental focus.

Individual Variability and Adaptation:

Individual variability and adaptation are essential considerations when undertaking a low-carb diet. It's crucial to understand that responses to such dietary changes can vary widely among individuals. Some may feel an immediate surge in energy, while others may go through an adaptation period as the body transitions to fat metabolism. Patience and a gradual approach to dietary changes are key factors in allowing the body to adapt and optimize energy production.

One of the distinctive features of the low-carb lifestyle is its ability to elicit diverse responses from individuals. While some may experience an instant boost in energy levels, others may initially undergo adjustments as the body adapts to the shift in fuel sources. This variability is influenced by factors such as metabolic rate, pre-existing dietary habits, overall health status, and individual biochemistry.

For individuals who have predominantly relied on carbohydrates for energy, the transition to utilizing fats as a primary energy source may require an adjustment period. This adaptation phase can bring about what is commonly known as the "keto flu," encompassing symptoms like fatigue, headaches, and irritability. It's important to note that these symptoms are typically temporary and often signal the body's adaptation to the metabolic shift.

Patience plays a key role during this adaptation phase, as the body needs time to optimize its energy production mechanisms. Gradual dietary changes, rather than sudden shifts, can facilitate a smoother transition and minimize potential discomfort. This approach allows individuals to adapt at their own pace, promoting a more sustainable integration of the low-carb lifestyle.

Additionally, it's crucial to recognize the personalized nature of dietary responses. What proves effective for one person may not yield the same results for another. Monitoring one's body and paying attention to signals such as energy levels, mood, and overall well-being can offer valuable insights into how an individual is responding to a low-carb diet.

Furthermore, seeking guidance from healthcare professionals or registered dietitians can provide personalized advice tailored to individual health considerations and goals. This collaborative approach ensures that dietary choices align with individual needs, promoting overall well-being.

While some individuals may notice immediate benefits, others might undergo an adaptation period during the shift to a low-carb lifestyle. Patience and a gradual approach are crucial in allowing the body to adapt to the metabolic shift, optimizing energy production, and contributing to the long-term success and sustainability of the low-carb lifestyle.

In conclusion, the increased energy levels associated with a low-carb lifestyle underscore the body's remarkable ability to adapt and thrive on alternative fuel sources. Prioritizing nutrient-dense foods, stabilizing blood sugar levels, and leveraging the benefits of fat metabolism empower individuals on a low-carb journey to unlock sustained vitality and experience heightened energy levels in their daily lives.

Crafting Balance: The Art of Building a Nutrient-Rich Low-Carb Diet

Crafting a balanced low-carb diet is a thoughtful endeavor that requires careful attention to nutrient composition, portion control, and individual preferences. While the primary focus is on reducing carbohydrate intake, achieving a well-rounded and sustainable dietary approach involves strategically choosing nutrient-dense foods that cater to individual needs. Here are key principles to guide the creation of a balanced low-carb diet.

Embrace Nutrient-Dense Foods:

Embracing nutrient-dense foods is a fundamental principle of a balanced low-carb diet, emphasizing the importance of choosing foods that are rich in essential nutrients. This dietary approach prioritizes whole, unprocessed options, including non-starchy vegetables, leafy greens, lean proteins, healthy fats, and, in moderation, low-sugar fruits. These nutrient-dense foods not only supply the body with crucial vitamins and minerals but also play a pivotal role in promoting satiety, curbing cravings, and supporting overall well-being.

Non-starchy Vegetables and Leafy Greens:

- Non-starchy vegetables and leafy greens are prominent components of a nutrient-dense low-carb diet. They are rich in fiber, vitamins, and minerals while being relatively low in carbohydrates. Examples include broccoli, cauliflower, spinach, kale, and bell peppers. These vegetables not only contribute to overall nutrient intake but also add color, flavor, and texture to meals.

Lean Proteins:

- Lean proteins, such as poultry, fish, tofu, and legumes, are essential for maintaining muscle mass and supporting various bodily functions. These protein sources are not only low in carbohydrates but also provide important amino acids necessary for optimal health. Including lean proteins in the diet helps promote satiety, contributing to a feeling of fullness and reducing the likelihood of overeating.

Healthy Fats:

- Healthy fats, such as those found in avocados, nuts, seeds, and olive oil, are integral to a balanced low-carb diet. These fats are not only nutrient-dense but also contribute to satiety and flavor in meals. Healthy fats play a role in supporting cognitive function, hormone production, and the absorption of fat-soluble vitamins.

Low-Sugar Fruits in Moderation:

- While fruits contain natural sugars, incorporating them in moderation provides essential vitamins and antioxidants. Berries, for instance, are lower in sugar compared to tropical fruits. Choosing fruits with a lower glycemic index can help manage blood sugar levels while still satisfying sweet cravings.

The emphasis on nutrient-dense foods aligns with the broader goal of nourishing the body with the essential building blocks for optimal health. These foods not only provide the necessary nutrients for various physiological functions but also support overall well-being by contributing to feelings of satisfaction and fullness.

By incorporating a variety of nutrient-dense foods, individuals following a low-carb diet can create well-rounded and satisfying meals. This approach not only addresses the macronutrient composition of the diet but also ensures that the body receives a diverse range of micronutrients, promoting a comprehensive and balanced nutritional profile.

Prioritize Lean Proteins

Prioritizing lean proteins is a fundamental aspect of a balanced low-carb diet, recognizing the pivotal role that protein plays in maintaining overall health. Protein serves as a critical component for maintaining muscle mass, supporting metabolic function, and promoting satiety. Opting for lean protein sources, such as poultry, fish, eggs, tofu, and legumes, aligns with the principles of a low-carb lifestyle, ensuring a high-quality protein intake without an excessive calorie or carbohydrate load.

Muscle Mass Maintenance:

- Lean proteins are essential for maintaining and building muscle mass. Muscle tissue plays a crucial role in overall metabolic health and contributes to the body's ability to burn calories efficiently. Prioritizing lean protein sources in a low-carb diet supports muscle preservation, especially when coupled with regular physical activity.

Metabolic Support:

- Protein is not only a building block for muscles but also plays a vital role in various metabolic processes. It aids in the synthesis of enzymes and hormones, contributing to the efficient functioning of the body's metabolic pathways. By prioritizing lean proteins, individuals can support these metabolic functions while adhering to the carbohydrate moderation characteristic of a low-carb lifestyle.

Feeling Full and Managing Hunger:

- One of the key advantages of incorporating lean proteins is their ability to promote a sense of fullness. Protein-rich foods tend to be more filling, helping individuals feel satisfied and reducing the likelihood of overeating. This aspect is particularly beneficial in weight management and aligns with the satiety-focused approach of a low-carb diet.

Additional Nutrients without Excessive Calories:

- Lean protein sources offer not only high-quality protein but also a range of additional nutrients. Poultry, fish, eggs, tofu, and legumes provide essential vitamins and minerals, contributing to overall nutritional balance. Importantly, these options deliver nutrients without an excessive calorie or carbohydrate load, allowing individuals to meet their protein needs while adhering to the principles of carbohydrate moderation.

By prioritizing lean proteins, individuals following a low-carb diet can craft meals that are not only satisfying but also nutritionally rich. Incorporating a variety of lean protein sources ensures a diverse array of essential amino acids and nutrients, contributing to a well-rounded and balanced dietary profile.

Incorporate Healthy Fats

Incorporating healthy fats is a fundamental component of a balanced low-carb diet, dispelling common misconceptions about the role of fats in a healthy eating plan. Opting for sources of healthy fats, such as avocados, nuts, seeds, olive oil, and fatty fish, is integral to the principles of a low-carb lifestyle. These sources not only provide essential fatty acids but also support brain health and contribute to a feeling of fullness. Balancing fat intake ensures a well-rounded approach to energy provision, particularly in the absence of high carbohydrate intake.

Essential Fatty Acids:

- Healthy fats are rich in essential fatty acids, such as omega-3 and omega-6 fatty acids. These play crucial roles in various physiological functions, including maintaining cell structure, supporting immune function, and contributing to cardiovascular health. Incorporating sources like fatty fish (rich in omega-3s), nuts, and seeds into a low-carb diet ensures the intake of these essential nutrients.

Brain Health Support:

- Fats are vital for brain health, as the brain is composed largely of fatty tissue. Healthy fats, especially those found in fatty fish, contribute to cognitive function and may have neuroprotective effects. The inclusion of these fats in a low-carb diet aligns with the holistic approach to well-being, recognizing the interconnectedness of nutrition and cognitive health.

Satiety and Fullness:

- Dietary fats contribute significantly to satiety, helping individuals feel full and satisfied after meals. This aspect is particularly beneficial in a low-carb context, where the reduction in carbohydrate intake may require compensation from other macronutrients to ensure a sense of fullness. Including healthy fats in meals supports this satiety-focused approach, aiding in portion control and overall adherence to the low-carb lifestyle.

Energy Provision in the Absence of High Carbohydrates:

- In a low-carb diet, where the traditional energy source of carbohydrates is moderated, fats become a primary energy provider. The body shifts to utilizing fats for fuel, a metabolic state known as ketosis. Healthy fats provide a sustained and efficient source of energy, helping individuals maintain energy levels throughout the day without the energy crashes associated with high-carbohydrate meals.

By incorporating a variety of healthy fats, individuals can create flavorful and satisfying meals that align with the principles of a low-carb lifestyle. From drizzling olive oil over salads to including avocados in meals, these sources not only enhance taste but also contribute to the overall nutritional profile of the diet.

In conclusion, recognizing the significance of incorporating healthy fats into a low-carb diet reflects a nuanced understanding of their crucial role in sustaining overall health. Whether it's supporting brain function, promoting a feeling of fullness, or serving as a primary energy source, healthy fats contribute to a comprehensive nutritional approach within the framework of carbohydrate moderation. This focus on the quality of nutrition ensures that those adhering to a low-carb lifestyle can embrace a diverse and fulfilling array of foods while successfully achieving their dietary objectives.

Include Non-Starchy Vegetables

Incorporating non-starchy vegetables is a fundamental element of a well-rounded low-carb diet, acknowledging the nutritional value and adaptability that these vegetables offer to meals. Non-starchy vegetables are notable for their abundance of fiber, vitamins, and minerals, making them a nutrient-dense option with Low-Carbohydrate content. Including a variety of colorful vegetables, such as leafy greens, broccoli, cauliflower, zucchini, and bell peppers, not only elevates the nutritional richness of meals but also adds visual appeal to the plate, creating a satisfying and wholesome dining experience.

Rich in Fiber, Vitamins, and Minerals:

- Non-starchy vegetables are excellent sources of dietary fiber, essential for digestive health and promoting a feeling of fullness. Additionally, they are packed with vitamins and minerals, including vitamin C, potassium, and folate, contributing to overall well-being. The diverse range of nutrients found in non-starchy vegetables supports various physiological functions and adds valuable micronutrients to the diet.

Low in Carbohydrates:

- A key feature of non-starchy vegetables is their low-carbohydrate content. This aligns with the principles of a low-carb lifestyle, allowing individuals to enjoy a variety of vegetables without significantly impacting their carbohydrate intake. This is particularly beneficial for those focusing on blood sugar control, weight management, and overall metabolic health.

Colorful Array for Nutritional Diversity:

- Incorporating a variety of non-starchy vegetables ensures a colorful and diverse array of nutrients. Different colors often signify distinct phytonutrients, each with its unique health benefits. From the deep greens of spinach to the vibrant hues of bell peppers, this diversity not only enhances the visual appeal of meals but also provides a broad spectrum of antioxidants and other bioactive compounds.

Satisfying and Appealing Plate:

- Non-starchy vegetables contribute to the overall satisfaction of meals by adding texture, flavor, and vibrancy to the plate. Their versatility allows for creative and satisfying meal combinations, ensuring that individuals following a low-carb diet can enjoy a diverse and appealing range of dishes.

Incorporating non-starchy vegetables into meals allows individuals to construct a well-rounded and nutritionally rich eating plan. Whether in salads or stir-fries, these vegetables form the basis for a variety of flavorful and gratifying dishes. Prioritizing non-starchy vegetables aligns with the broader objective of promoting a balanced and sustainable nutritional approach within the framework of a low-carb lifestyle.

Apart from their Low-Carbohydrate content, these vegetables offer a plethora of nutrients, contribute to meal satisfaction, and enhance the visual appeal of the plate. This emphasis on nutritional diversity ensures that individuals can relish a satisfying and healthful array of foods while adhering to the principles of carbohydrate moderation.

Monitor Portion Sizes

Keeping an eye on portion sizes is a crucial element of sustaining a balanced low-carb diet, highlighting the significance of mindful eating even when opting for nutrient-dense foods. While the emphasis is on the quality of selected foods, controlling portions is essential in averting the intake of excess calories. Grasping individual energy requirements and adapting portion sizes accordingly is vital for attaining and preserving weight management objectives. This practice is fundamental for fostering overall health and well-being within the context of a low-carb lifestyle.

Balancing Nutrient Density with Portion Control:

- Nutrient-dense foods are central to a low-carb diet, providing essential vitamins, minerals, and other beneficial compounds. However, even with healthier choices, consuming excessive portions can contribute to an imbalance in caloric intake. Monitoring portion sizes ensures that individuals derive the nutritional benefits of these foods without exceeding their energy requirements.

Preventing Overconsumption of Calories:

- Portion control acts as a safeguard against overconsumption of calories, which is crucial for weight management. Even when opting for nutrient-dense options, an excess of calories can hinder progress toward health and wellness goals. Being mindful of portion sizes allows individuals to strike a balance between enjoying satisfying meals and maintaining an appropriate caloric intake.

Individualized Approach to Energy Needs:

- Each person has unique energy requirements based on factors such as age, activity level, and metabolic rate. Monitoring portion sizes involves recognizing and adapting to these individual needs. Tailoring serving sizes according to one's energy expenditure ensures that the body receives an appropriate amount of fuel while aligning with the principles of a low-carb lifestyle.

Key to Achieving and Sustaining Weight Management Goals:

- Portion control is a key factor in achieving and sustaining weight management goals. By avoiding excessive calorie intake, individuals can contribute to weight loss or maintenance within the context of a low-carb diet. This practice supports a holistic approach to health, where both the quality and quantity of food are considered integral components.

Mindful Eating Practices:

- Monitoring portion sizes promotes mindful eating, encouraging individuals to be present and intentional during meals. This practice involves paying attention to hunger and fullness cues, savoring each bite, and cultivating a greater awareness of the overall eating experience. Mindful eating aligns with the principles of Carb Conscious Living, fostering a positive relationship with food.

In conclusion, focusing on nutrient-dense options remains essential in a low-carb diet, yet paying careful attention to portion sizes is equally vital. This strategy guarantees that individuals find harmony between relishing flavorful and gratifying meals while adhering to an appropriate caloric intake. The inclusion of portion control, as part of the broader Carbo-Conscious Living approach, plays a role in attaining and preserving weight management objectives, fostering overall well-being.

Strategically Choose Carbohydrates

Making wise choices regarding carbohydrates is a key element of an informed low-carb lifestyle. This involves not only reducing overall carbohydrate intake but also assessing the quality and effects of the carbohydrates chosen. Prioritizing complex carbohydrates with a lower glycemic index is essential for sustaining a balanced nutritional approach in the context of a low-carb diet. This strategic preference encompasses whole grains, legumes, and low-sugar fruits, providing lasting energy without causing pronounced spikes in blood sugar levels.

Reducing Overall Carbohydrate Intake:

- The primary focus of a low-carb lifestyle is the conscious reduction of overall carbohydrate intake. This is based on the understanding that excessive carbohydrates, especially those with a high glycemic index, can lead to fluctuations in blood sugar levels and impact metabolic health. By moderating carbohydrate intake, individuals aim to achieve better blood sugar control and support overall well-being.

Strategic Choices within the Carbohydrate Category:

- Strategic carbohydrate choices involve discerning between different types of carbohydrates based on their impact on blood sugar levels. Rather than eliminating carbohydrates, the emphasis is on selecting complex carbohydrates, which are slower to digest and have a lower glycemic index. This nuanced approach recognizes that not all carbohydrates are equal and that their quality matters in the context of a low-carb lifestyle.

Opting for Complex Carbohydrates:

- Complex carbohydrates, found in whole grains, legumes, and certain fruits, are characterized by their more complex molecular structure. This complexity results in a slower rate of digestion and absorption, providing a gradual and sustained release of glucose into the bloodstream. Choosing these types of carbohydrates helps prevent rapid spikes in blood sugar, supporting stable energy levels throughout the day.

- Here is a list of foods that contain complex carbohydrates:

- Whole Grains:

  - Brown rice

  - Quinoa

  - Barley

  - Oats (e.g., old-fashioned oats, steel-cut oats)

- Legumes:

  - Lentils

- ○ Chickpeas

- ○ Black beans

- ○ Kidney beans

- Vegetables:

  - ○ Sweet potatoes

  - ○ Butternut squash

  - ○ Peas

  - ○ Broccoli

- Whole Fruits:

  - ○ Apples

  - ○ Berries (e.g., blueberries, strawberries)

  - ○ Oranges

  - ○ Pears

- Whole Grain Products:

  - ○ Whole wheat bread

  - ○ Whole grain pasta

  - ○ Whole grain cereal

  - ○ Quinoa pasta

  - ○ Nuts and Seeds:

  - ○ Almonds

- Walnuts

- Chia seeds

- Flaxseeds

Incorporating these complex carbohydrates into your diet can contribute to sustained energy levels and overall health.

Lower Glycemic Index Choices:

- The glycemic index (GI) is a measure of how quickly a carbohydrate-containing food raises blood sugar levels. Low GI foods are associated with a slower and steadier increase in blood glucose. By opting for carbohydrates with a lower glycemic index, individuals on a low-carb diet can enjoy the benefits of sustained energy without the abrupt fluctuations that can affect insulin sensitivity and overall metabolic health.

- Here is a list of foods with lower glycemic indexes:

- Legumes:

  - Lentils

  - Chickpeas

  - Black beans

  - Kidney beans

- Whole Grains:

  - Quinoa

  - Barley

- o Steel-cut oats

- o Whole wheat products (e.g., bread, pasta)

- Non-Starchy Vegetables:

  - o Broccoli

  - o Cauliflower

  - o Spinach

  - o Zucchini

- Sweet Potatoes:

  - o Sweet potatoes have a lower GI compared to regular potatoes.

- Most Fruits:

  - o Berries (e.g., strawberries, blueberries)

  - o Cherries

  - o Apples

  - o Pears

- Nuts and Seeds:

  - o Almonds

  - o Walnuts

  - o Chia seeds

  - o Flaxseeds

- Dairy Products:

- ○ Whole milk

- ○ Yogurt (unsweetened, plain)

- Pasta:

  - ○ Whole wheat pasta

  - ○ Pasta cooked al dente (firm to the bite)

- Bulgar:

  - ○ Bulgur wheat

- Barley:

  - ○ Barley grains

Remember that the glycemic index can be influenced by various factors, including food combinations and preparation methods. It's also important to consider portion sizes and overall meal composition for better blood sugar management.

Providing Sustained Energy:

- The strategic choice of carbohydrates in a low-carb lifestyle ensures that individuals receive sustained energy from their dietary sources. This is particularly important for maintaining energy levels throughout the day, supporting physical activities, and avoiding the energy crashes associated with high-glycemic carbohydrates.

In conclusion, making wise choices about carbohydrates requires careful consideration of the types of carbs we consume. When selecting complex carbohydrates with a lower glycemic index, those following a low-carb lifestyle can reap the nutritional rewards of these foods. Not only does this contribute to stable blood sugar levels, but it also provides a lasting source of energy. This approach is in harmony with the principles of Carbo-Conscious Living, highlighting the importance of making thoughtful and strategic dietary decisions to support overall health and well-being.

Hydration

In a balanced low-carb diet, staying hydrated is a key element, underscoring the significance of maintaining sufficient fluid intake for overall health and well-being. Water, an essential resource for various bodily functions, is crucial for supporting digestion, nutrient absorption, and temperature regulation. In the context of a low-carb lifestyle, prioritizing hydration becomes essential for optimizing physiological processes without relying on sugary beverages. Important considerations for staying well-hydrated in the context of a low-carb framework include.

The Essential Role of Water in Bodily Functions:

- Water is indispensable for various physiological functions, including the digestion and absorption of nutrients. It serves as a medium for chemical reactions in the body, aids in the transportation of nutrients, and helps regulate body temperature through sweating and respiration. Adequate hydration is vital for maintaining optimal bodily functions.

Supporting Digestion and Nutrient Absorption:

- Proper hydration is integral to the digestive process. Water facilitates the breakdown of food in the stomach, supports the absorption of nutrients in the intestines, and aids in the elimination of waste products. Ensuring sufficient hydration promotes efficient digestion and nutrient utilization.

Temperature Regulation:

- Hydration plays a crucial role in regulating body temperature, particularly through the cooling effect of sweating. This becomes especially relevant during physical activities or in warmer environments. Maintaining proper hydration levels supports the body's ability to cool itself, preventing issues such as dehydration and heat-related illnesses.

Flavoring Water Without Added Sugars:

- In a low-carb diet, where the focus is on reducing sugar intake, it's important to find ways to add flavor to water without resorting to sugary beverages. Infusing water with natural flavors such as citrus slices, herbs, or cucumber provides a refreshing and enjoyable alternative. This enhances the palatability of water without compromising the principles of Carb Conscious Living.

Avoiding Sugary Beverages:

- Sugary beverages, commonly associated with high-carbohydrate content, are not in alignment with the low-carb lifestyle. These beverages can contribute to excessive calorie intake, blood sugar spikes, and other health issues. Choosing water as the primary source of hydration supports the principles of a low-carb diet by ensuring a calorie-free, sugar-free option.

- Diet soft drinks, which are typically sugar-free and low in carbohydrates, can be considered acceptable as part of a low-carb lifestyle. However, it's important to note that while they don't contain sugar, they often use sugar substitutes or artificial sweeteners to achieve sweetness. Some people may prefer to avoid artificial sweeteners for various reasons.

- Individual responses to artificial sweeteners can vary, and some people may experience cravings, digestive issues, or other reactions. If you tolerate artificial sweeteners well and they don't negatively impact your health or cravings, incorporating diet soft drinks in moderation may be acceptable for you within a low-carb lifestyle.

- It's advisable to be mindful of your body's response to diet soft drinks and to consider other hydration options, such as water, herbal teas, or naturally flavored water, to maintain optimal health and well-being.

- Individualized Hydration Needs:

- Hydration needs vary among individuals based on factors such as age, activity level, and climate. Tailoring fluid intake to individual requirements ensures that each person meets their specific hydration needs for optimal health and performance.

Emphasizing water as the primary source of hydration aligns with the principles of Carbo-Conscious Living by avoiding the pitfalls associated with sugary beverages. Infusing water with natural flavors provides a delightful way to enhance taste without compromising the health-conscious approach of a low-carb diet. Hydration, when approached mindfully, contributes to overall well-being and complements the holistic focus on health within the low-carb framework.

Individualized Approaches

In summary, embracing individualized approaches is a fundamental principle of a well-considered low-carb lifestyle, understanding that the notion of balance is subjective and differs from person to person. It's essential to acknowledge and honor these individual variations, allowing for the customization of the low-carb diet to align with specific requirements. This involves making adaptations based on factors like activity levels, health objectives, and personal likes and dislikes. The following key points highlight the importance of personalized strategies within the framework of a low-carb lifestyle:

Subjectivity of Balance:

- Balance, especially in the context of a diet, is a subjective concept. What constitutes a balanced approach to nutrition can vary widely among individuals based on their unique circumstances, goals, and preferences. Acknowledging this subjectivity is the first step toward developing an individualized approach to the low-carb lifestyle.

Factors Influencing Individual Needs:

- Various factors influence the dietary needs of individuals, including their level of physical activity, specific health goals, and personal preferences. Someone engaged in intense physical training may have different energy requirements than a sedentary individual. Likewise, someone managing a specific health condition may need to tailor their low-carb approach to address those considerations.

Tailoring to Energy Requirements:

- Individual energy requirements differ based on factors such as age, gender, metabolism, and activity level. Tailoring the low-carb diet to suit these energy needs ensures that individuals receive an appropriate amount of fuel for their daily activities, supporting both physical performance and overall well-being.

Dietary Tolerances and Preferences:

- Each person has unique tolerances and preferences when it comes to food. Some individuals may have specific dietary restrictions or intolerances, while others may have personal preferences that influence their food choices. An individualized low-carb approach considers these factors, allowing for flexibility and enjoyment in food selection.

Lifestyle Considerations:

- Lifestyle factors, such as work schedule, social commitments, and culinary skills, play a significant role in determining the practicality and sustainability of a low-carb diet. Recognizing these lifestyle considerations helps individuals make realistic and feasible adjustments to their dietary choices.

Gradual Adjustments and Flexibility:

- Individualized approaches involve a process of gradual adjustments and flexibility. It may take time to find the right balance that aligns with individual goals and preferences. Being open to experimentation and making informed adjustments allows for a sustainable and enjoyable low-carb lifestyle.

Monitoring and Adapting:

- Regular monitoring of progress and an ongoing assessment of how the low-carb approach aligns with individual goals are essential. This involves staying attuned to changes in energy levels, weight management, and overall well-being. If necessary, individuals can adapt their approach based on evolving needs and circumstances.

Customizing the low-carb diet to meet individual needs, taking into account factors like energy demands, dietary preferences, and lifestyle choices, empowers individuals to establish a personalized and enduring approach to health and nutrition. This approach aligns with the principles of Carbo-Conscious Living, highlighting a mindful and adaptable journey toward well-being.

In conclusion, achieving a balanced low-carb diet requires a thoughtful blend of nutrient-dense foods, portion management, and personalized choices. Through the inclusion of a variety of whole foods, careful monitoring of portion sizes, and the incorporation of strategic carbohydrates, individuals can create a sustainable and nourishing dietary approach that resonates with their health and wellness objectives.

Meal Planning and Preparation: A Blueprint for Success

Planning and preparing meals play vital roles in the success and sustainability of a low-carb lifestyle. In exploring this crucial aspect, we'll delve into incorporating lean proteins and healthy fats into weekly meal plans, providing diverse ideas for breakfast, lunch, dinner, and snacks. Furthermore, we'll offer sample recipes that embody the principles of a well-balanced low-carb diet. To streamline the process, we'll discuss the efficiency of batch cooking and share valuable tips for effective meal preparation.

When considering weekly meal plans, breakfast options may include Greek yogurt with berries and a sprinkle of nuts, a spinach and feta omelet, or chia seed pudding with almond milk and sliced strawberries. For lunch, think about a grilled chicken salad with mixed greens, cherry tomatoes, and avocado, zucchini noodles with shrimp and pesto sauce, or turkey and vegetable lettuce wraps. Dinner selections could involve baked salmon with lemon and dill, accompanied by roasted Brussels sprouts, cauliflower crust pizza with assorted vegetable toppings, or stir-fried tofu with broccoli, bell peppers, and a sesame ginger sauce. Snack choices might include cheese and cucumber slices, almond butter on celery sticks, or hard-boiled eggs with a dash of salt.

As for sample recipes, a grilled chicken Caesar salad could be prepared by tossing grilled chicken and vegetables with Caesar dressing for a satisfying and protein-rich meal. Alternatively, cauliflower fried rice could be made by stir-frying cauliflower rice with diced vegetables (carrots, peas, bell peppers) and scrambled eggs, seasoned with soy sauce for a low-carb alternative to traditional fried rice.

In terms of meal preparation tips, batch cooking is a time-saving strategy involving the preparation of larger quantities of meals that are portioned for future consumption. An example of this would be cooking a large batch of grilled chicken, roast vegetables, and quinoa on the weekend and portioning them into containers for quick and convenient lunches throughout the week. Additionally, efficient meal prep involves designating a specific day for meal prep, planning meals with common ingredients to minimize waste, investing in quality storage containers, pre-cutting vegetables, marinating proteins, and organizing ingredients in advance for seamless cooking sessions. Embracing variety and flexibility in weekly meal plans ensures a diverse nutrient intake and prevents monotony, allowing for adjustments in portion sizes and ingredients based on individual preferences and nutritional needs. Ultimately, mastering the art of meal planning and preparation enhances the feasibility of sustaining a nutrient-rich and flavorful low-carb diet.

Quick and Easy Low Carb Recipes: Culinary Delights in Minutes

Navigating a low-carb lifestyle doesn't mean sacrificing flavor or spending endless hours in the kitchen. In fact, a plethora of quick and easy low-carb recipes exist, ensuring that delicious and nutritious meals can be prepared with minimal effort. Let's explore a couple of mouthwatering options that exemplify the simplicity and creativity inherent in low-carb cooking.

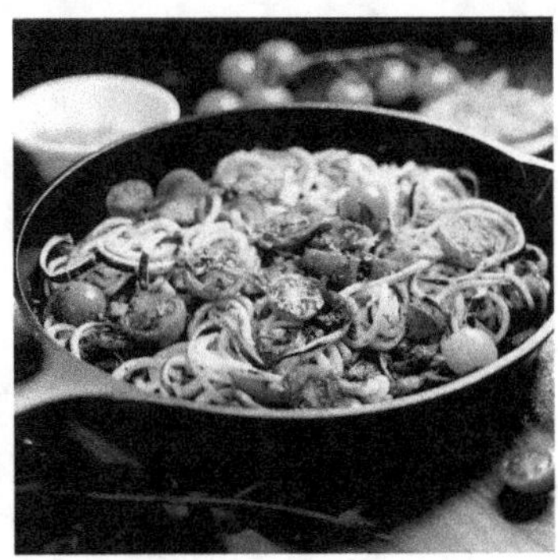

- **Zucchini Noodles with Pesto and Cherry Tomatoes:**

- *Ingredients:*

  - 2 medium-sized zucchinis (spiralized into noodles)

  - 1 cup cherry tomatoes (halved)

  - 1/4 cup fresh basil pesto

  - 2 tablespoons grated Parmesan cheese

  - Salt and pepper to taste

- *Instructions:*

  - In a pan over medium heat, sauté zucchini noodles until tender (approximately 2-3 minutes).

  - Toss in cherry tomatoes and cook for an additional 1-2 minutes.

  - Remove from heat and stir in fresh basil pesto.

  - Garnish with grated Parmesan cheese, salt, and pepper. Serve warm.

- Avocado and Egg Salad Lettuce Wraps:

  - *Ingredients:*

    - 2 avocados (diced)

    - 4 hard-boiled eggs (chopped)

    - 1/4 cup red onion (finely diced)

    - 2 tablespoons mayonnaise

    - 1 tablespoon Dijon mustard

- Salt and pepper to taste

- Butter lettuce leaves (for wrapping)

○ *Instructions:*

- In a bowl, combine diced avocados, chopped hard-boiled eggs, red onion, mayonnaise, and Dijon mustard.

- Mix until ingredients are well combined. Season with salt and pepper to taste.

- Spoon the mixture onto butter lettuce leaves, creating wraps.

- Enjoy the refreshing and satisfying avocado and egg salad wraps.

These recipes not only showcase the diversity of flavors achievable with minimal ingredients but also underscore the adaptability of Low-Carb cooking. The simplicity of zucchini noodles with pesto and cherry tomatoes provides a vibrant and pasta-like experience without the carb overload. On the other hand, the avocado and egg salad lettuce wraps offer a satisfying combination of creamy textures and savory notes, all while keeping carbohydrate content in check.

The beauty of quick and easy low-carb recipes lies in their accessibility for individuals with various culinary skill levels and time constraints. These recipes serve as a testament to the fact that embracing a low-carb lifestyle can be both delicious and convenient, ensuring that the journey toward health is as enjoyable as it is nourishing.

See more recipes in the Appendix to our book.

Staying Active on a Low-Carb Lifestyle: A Holistic Approach to Well-Being

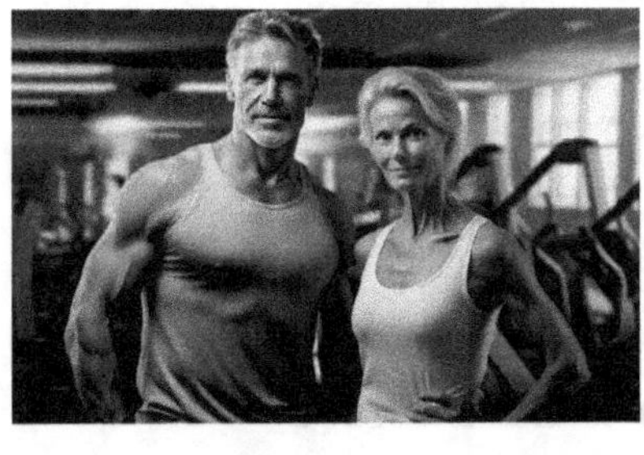

Sustaining an active lifestyle is a crucial and non-negotiable element of a comprehensive approach to well-being within the context of a low-carb lifestyle. Beyond the focus on dietary decisions, the importance of physical activity cannot be emphasized enough, as it profoundly influences metabolism and contributes to overall health. Regular exercise directly and in various ways affects metabolic processes, improving the body's efficiency in utilizing nutrients and aligning with the principles of a low-carb diet. Here are key points to delve into this topic:

Holistic Well-Being:

- A holistic approach to well-being encompasses more than just dietary choices. It integrates various lifestyle factors, with physical activity being a cornerstone. By adopting an active lifestyle, individuals contribute to their overall health and vitality, aligning with the comprehensive goals of a low-carb lifestyle.

Impact on Metabolism:

- Consistent physical activity directly impacts metabolic processes, improving the efficiency of energy utilization. This enhancement promotes the effective breakdown of nutrients, especially those obtained from a low-carb diet. The symbiotic connection between regular exercise and metabolism plays a pivotal role in reaching and sustaining health-related objectives.

Efficient Nutrient Utilization:

- Physical activity enhances the body's ability to efficiently utilize nutrients, ensuring that the energy derived from a low-carb diet is optimally utilized. This efficiency supports various metabolic functions, including the utilization of fats for energy, a key aspect of low-carb living.

Supporting the Principles of a Low-Carb Diet:

- Regular exercise complements and reinforces the principles of a low-carb diet. It contributes to weight management by burning calories and promoting lean muscle mass.

Enhanced Insulin Sensitivity:

- Exercise plays a pivotal role in enhancing insulin sensitivity, which is particularly relevant for individuals following a low-carb lifestyle. Improved insulin sensitivity allows for more effective regulation of blood sugar levels, reducing the risk of insulin resistance and related health issues.

Contributing to Overall Health:

- Physical activity is not only about weight management but also about promoting overall health. Regular exercise has been associated with cardiovascular health, improved mental well-being, and a reduced risk of chronic diseases. This holistic approach aligns with the broader goals of well-rounded health within the context of a low-carb lifestyle.

Sustainable Well-Being:

- Incorporating physical activity into a low-carb lifestyle is not just a short-term strategy but a commitment to sustained well-being. Regular exercise contributes to increased energy levels, better mood, and enhanced cognitive function, fostering a sense of vitality that goes hand-in-hand with the principles of Carb Conscious Living.

Maintaining an active lifestyle is an integral aspect of a holistic approach to well-being within the framework of a low-carb lifestyle. Regular exercise impacts metabolism, enhances nutrient utilization, and supports the principles of a low-carb diet, contributing to both short-term and long-term health goals. By recognizing the importance of physical activity, individuals can create a synergistic relationship between their dietary choices and their overall lifestyle, leading to a more comprehensive and sustainable approach to health and well-being.

The significance of physical activity extends far beyond its metabolic benefits; it plays a crucial and multi-faceted role in sustaining a positive mindset and fostering emotional well-being. Recognizing the interconnectedness of physical and mental health, finding enjoyable workouts tailored to personal preferences is pivotal. This ensures that exercise becomes a gratifying and sustainable aspect of daily life, contributing not only to physical health but also to emotional and mental wellness. Here are key points to elaborate on this theme:

Holistic Well-Being:

- Physical activity is an integral component of holistic well-being, encompassing both physical and mental dimensions. The connection between exercise and emotional health is profound, with regular activity contributing to a positive mindset and overall emotional well-being.

Positive Impact on Mood:

- Engaging in physical activity triggers the release of endorphins, often referred to as "feel-good" hormones. These biochemical responses have a direct impact on mood regulation, promoting feelings of happiness, relaxation, and a sense of well-being. This positive influence is vital for maintaining emotional balance.

Stress Reduction:

- Physical activity serves as a powerful tool for stress reduction. Whether it's the rhythmic movements of jogging, the mindfulness of yoga, or the adrenaline rush of cycling, exercise helps alleviate stress by promoting relaxation and providing an outlet for pent-up tension.

Tailoring Workouts to Personal Preferences:

- Personalizing the choice of workouts based on individual preferences is essential. Whether someone finds joy in dancing, tranquility in yoga, or exhilaration in hiking, aligning physical activity with personal interests ensures that exercise is not perceived as a chore but as a rewarding and enjoyable experience.

Gratification and Sustainability:

- The key to sustaining an active lifestyle is to discover activities that bring joy and satisfaction. When exercise is enjoyable, individuals are more likely to integrate it into their daily routines consistently. This transformation from a routine to a rewarding experience enhances the gratification derived from physical activity.

Diverse Options for Enjoyable Workouts:

- The range of enjoyable workouts is vast, allowing individuals to explore various activities until they find what resonates with them. Whether it's group classes, outdoor activities, or home-based routines, diverse options ensure that everyone can discover a form of exercise that suits their preferences and lifestyle.

Positive Impact on Self-Esteem:

- Regular physical activity positively influences self-esteem and body image. Achieving personal fitness goals, regardless of size or intensity, contributes to a sense of accomplishment and boosts self-confidence. This positive reinforcement extends beyond the workout session, influencing how individuals perceive themselves in daily life.

Transforming Exercise into a Rewarding Experience:

- The ultimate goal is to transform exercise from a perceived obligation into a rewarding experience. This shift in mindset contributes to the sustainability of an active lifestyle, making it a lifelong commitment rather than a short-term endeavor.

By tailoring workouts to personal preferences and discovering activities that bring joy, individuals can make exercise a gratifying and sustainable aspect of their daily lives. This holistic approach recognizes the interconnectedness of physical and emotional health, promoting a balanced and fulfilling lifestyle.

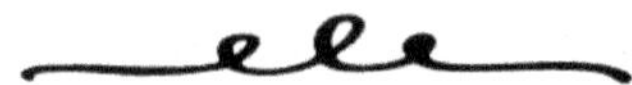

Incorporating exercise into daily life is a fundamental and indispensable aspect of a balanced low-carb lifestyle. Recognizing the challenges posed by busy schedules, strategic planning and creative solutions become pivotal in making regular physical activity not only attainable but an integral part of one's routine. Employing various strategies, such as scheduling workouts, opting for active commuting, and integrating short bursts of activity throughout the day, contributes to a cumulative and effective approach to staying active, even amidst a hectic lifestyle. Here are key points to elaborate on this theme:

Strategic Planning for Busy Schedules:

- Busy schedules often pose a significant barrier to regular exercise. Strategic planning involves proactively scheduling dedicated time for workouts, treating them with the same priority as other essential commitments. This intentional approach ensures that exercise becomes a non-negotiable part of the daily routine.

Calendar Integration for Workouts:

- Scheduling workouts into daily calendars is an effective strategy to create a structured and consistent exercise routine. By allocating specific time slots for physical activity, individuals can better manage their time and overcome the challenges posed by a hectic schedule.

Active Commuting:

- For those with limited time for dedicated workouts, incorporating physical activity into daily commuting is a practical solution. Opting for active commuting, such as walking or cycling to work, not only saves time but also adds a regular dose of exercise to the daily routine.

Short Bursts of Activity Throughout the Day:

- Breaking down exercise into shorter, more manageable bursts throughout the day is a creative solution for busy individuals. This can include taking short walks during breaks, doing quick bodyweight exercises, or incorporating stretches between tasks. Cumulatively, these short bursts contribute to the recommended daily physical activity.

Utilizing Technology for Reminders:

- Leveraging technology, such as fitness apps or reminders on smartphones, can serve as helpful tools in staying accountable to regular exercise. Setting reminders or alarms for scheduled workout times can prompt individuals to prioritize physical activity even amid a demanding schedule.

Workplace Movement Initiatives:

- Some workplaces encourage physical activity by implementing movement initiatives. This may include standing desks, walking meetings, or designated spaces for stretching and exercise. Such initiatives foster a workplace culture that values and supports the integration of movement into the daily routine.

Flexibility and Adaptability:

- Recognizing the dynamic nature of busy schedules, flexibility and adaptability are key. Individuals may need to adjust their workout times or routines based on changing demands. Embracing flexibility ensures that exercise remains achievable and sustainable in the long run.

Mindful Integration of Movement:

- Mindful integration involves being aware of opportunities for movement throughout the day. This could include taking the stairs instead of the elevator, parking farther away to encourage walking or incorporating physical activity during leisure time.

Cumulative Approach to Activity:

- Emphasizing a cumulative approach acknowledges the total amount of physical activity throughout a day matters. Short, frequent bouts of movement can add up to meet recommended activity levels, making it feasible for individuals with demanding schedules.

In summary, integrating exercise into daily routines while following a low-carb lifestyle demands thoughtful planning and inventive solutions. Whether it's through planned workout sessions, incorporating activity into daily commutes, or engaging in brief bursts of exercise, individuals can establish and sustain an active lifestyle, even amid busy schedules. The crucial factor is acknowledging the significance of physical activity and embracing adaptable strategies that resonate with personal preferences and accommodate lifestyle constraints.

The harmonious connection between a low-carb lifestyle and an active daily approach establishes the groundwork for holistic well-being. Acknowledging the significance of physical activity, considering its metabolic and emotional advantages, underscores the transformative power of a holistic health approach. Through the integration of enjoyable workouts and the adoption of creative strategies for staying active in busy schedules, individuals can fully embrace the symbiotic relationship between movement and a low-carb lifestyle.

Mindful Eating and Emotional Well-being: Nourishing the Body and Soul

In the context of a well-rounded and rewarding low-carb lifestyle, the concept of mindful eating becomes a foundational element for emotional well-being. Mindful eating transcends the mere act of choosing food; it encompasses a deliberate and conscious method of consuming our meals. By fostering a heightened awareness of the eating experience, individuals can establish a deeper connection with their food. This practice involves relishing every bite, recognizing the diverse flavors and textures in the food, and closely observing the body's responses throughout the meal. Here are key insights to delve into this concept:

Holistic Approach to Well-Being:

- Mindful eating is positioned as an integral aspect of a holistic approach to well-being within the context of a low-carb lifestyle. It emphasizes not only the nutritional content of the food but also the overall experience of eating, recognizing the interconnectedness of physical and emotional health.

Conscious Awareness of Eating Experience:

- At its core, mindful eating involves conscious awareness of the entire eating experience. This includes being present in the moment, fully engaged with the act of eating, and acknowledging the sensory aspects of the meal.

Savoring Each Bite:

- Mindful eaters take the time to savor each bite, appreciating the flavors, aromas, and textures of the food. This intentional approach allows individuals to derive maximum pleasure and satisfaction from their meals, transforming eating into a sensory-rich experience.

Appreciation of Flavors and Textures:

- An essential aspect of mindful eating is the appreciation of the diverse flavors and textures present in the food. This goes beyond mere consumption; it involves actively engaging with the sensory elements of the meal, fostering a deeper connection with the culinary experience.

Attentiveness to Body Responses:

- Mindful eaters pay close attention to their body's responses during the meal. This includes being attuned to hunger and fullness cues, as well as recognizing how different foods impact energy levels and overall well-being. This heightened awareness fosters a more intuitive and responsive approach to eating.

Preventing Emotional and Stress-Related Eating:

- Mindful eating serves as a protective measure against emotional and stress-related eating. By staying attuned to the present moment and focusing on the sensory aspects of the meal, individuals can avoid mindless or impulsive eating driven by emotions.

Enhancing Emotional Well-Being:

- The practice of mindful eating contributes to emotional well-being by fostering a positive relationship with food. It encourages a non-judgmental awareness of eating habits, promoting self-compassion and reducing the potential for negative emotions associated with food choices.

Cultivating Gratitude for Nourishment:

- Mindful eating involves cultivating gratitude for the nourishment provided by food. By acknowledging the effort and energy invested in producing and preparing meals, individuals develop a sense of appreciation and gratitude for the sustenance they receive.

Promoting Healthy Digestion:

- Beyond emotional well-being, mindful eating has been associated with promoting healthy digestion. Being present and focused during meals allows the body to enter a more relaxed state, optimizing the digestive process and nutrient absorption.

Through relishing every bite, acknowledging diverse flavors and textures, and tuning into the body's responses, individuals can cultivate a profound connection with their meals, enhancing emotional well-being in the context of a well-balanced low-carb lifestyle.

Central to mindful eating is the art of eating with awareness. This involves being fully present in the moment, devoid of distractions, and completely engaged in the act of eating. By immersing oneself in the sensory aspects of the meal, individuals can extract greater satisfaction from their food, nurturing a more fulfilling and nourishing relationship with the act of eating.

Listening to hunger and fullness cues is a crucial dimension of mindful eating that significantly contributes to emotional well-being within the context of a balanced low-carb lifestyle. This practice involves tuning in to the body's signals, allowing individuals to distinguish genuine hunger from emotional or external triggers. Here are key points on this aspect of mindful eating:

Empowerment through Awareness:

- Listening to hunger and fullness cues empowers individuals with a heightened sense of awareness regarding their body's needs. This awareness serves as a powerful tool in distinguishing between physical hunger and other non-nutritional factors that may drive eating behavior.

Distinguishing Genuine Hunger:

- Mindful eaters develop the ability to distinguish genuine hunger from emotional or external triggers. This skill is pivotal in preventing mindless or impulsive eating and ensures that food intake is driven by physiological needs rather than emotional responses.

Balanced and Intuitive Eating:

- The practice of tuning into hunger and fullness cues fosters a balanced and intuitive approach to eating. Individuals become more attuned to the natural rhythm of their body's hunger and satiety signals, allowing them to make conscious choices about when to start and stop eating.

Preventing Emotional Eating:

- Mindful eating, anchored in the awareness of hunger cues, acts as a preventative measure against emotional eating. By recognizing the emotional triggers that may prompt unnecessary eating, individuals can make informed decisions to address emotional needs without relying on food.

Aligning Nutritional Intake with Body's Rhythm:

- One of the key benefits of listening to hunger and fullness cues is the alignment of nutritional intake with the body's natural rhythm. This ensures that meals are initiated when the body genuinely requires nourishment and concludes when the body signals satisfaction, promoting a more harmonious relationship with food.

Enhancing Mind-Body Connection:

- The mindful practice of tuning into hunger and fullness cues enhances the mind-body connection. This connection is essential for developing a more profound understanding of how dietary choices impact overall well-being, both physically and emotionally.

Cultivating Intuitive Decision-Making:

- Mindful eaters cultivate intuitive decision-making around food. By listening to their body's signals, they are more likely to make choices aligned with their nutritional needs, leading to a sense of empowerment and control over their eating habits.

Reducing Guilt and Shame:

- The ability to listen to hunger and fullness cues also plays a role in reducing feelings of guilt and shame associated with eating. Individuals learn to trust their bodies, promoting a positive and non-judgmental relationship with food.

Mindful Choices for Sustained Well-Being:

- The practice of tuning into hunger and fullness cues supports individuals in making mindful choices that contribute to sustained well-being. This mindful approach extends beyond the immediate moment, fostering a long-term positive relationship with food.

Listening to hunger and fullness cues is a transformative dimension of mindful eating within a low-carb lifestyle. By distinguishing genuine hunger, preventing emotional eating, and aligning nutritional intake with the body's natural rhythm, individuals can foster emotional well-being and make conscious choices that contribute to their overall health and vitality.

Addressing emotional eating is a pivotal aspect of mindful eating within a low-carb lifestyle, requiring a thoughtful exploration of the psychological dimensions that influence our relationship with food. The following points elaborate on the importance of addressing emotional eating:

Psychological Dimensions of Eating:

- Emotional eating delves into the psychological aspects of our relationship with food. It acknowledges that eating is not solely driven by physiological hunger but is often influenced by emotions, stress, boredom, or other psychological factors.

Identification of Emotional Triggers:

- The first crucial step in addressing emotional eating is identifying the specific triggers that prompt such behavior. These triggers can vary widely, encompassing stress, boredom, loneliness, sadness, or even happiness. Recognizing these triggers is essential for gaining insight into the underlying emotional drivers of one's eating patterns.

Heightened Self-Awareness:

- The process of identifying emotional triggers cultivates heightened self-awareness. Individuals become more attuned to the emotional cues that precede or accompany their desire to eat. This increased awareness lays the foundation for making conscious and informed choices in response to emotional stimuli.

Informed Decision-Making:

- Armed with knowledge about their emotional triggers, individuals are better equipped to make informed decisions about how to respond to emotional cues. Rather than turning to food as an automatic response, they can explore alternative coping mechanisms or strategies to address the root cause of the emotional need.

Development of Coping Strategies:

- Addressing emotional eating involves the development of effective coping strategies. Whether through mindfulness practices, stress management techniques, or engaging in activities that bring joy and fulfillment, individuals can cultivate healthier ways to navigate and respond to emotional challenges without relying on food.

Breaking the Cycle:

- By identifying emotional triggers and developing alternative coping strategies, individuals can break the cycle of using food as a primary means of emotional regulation. This transformative process fosters a more balanced and intentional relationship with food, reducing reliance on emotional eating habits.

Mindful Response to Emotional Cues:

- Mindful eating encourages a deliberate and conscious response to emotional cues. Rather than seeking solace in food impulsively, individuals can apply mindfulness techniques to assess their emotional state, understand the source of discomfort, and choose responses that align with their overall well-being.

Prevention of Unconscious Eating:

- Addressing emotional eating also helps prevent unconscious or mindless eating. By recognizing emotional triggers, individuals can avoid the trap of consuming food without genuine hunger, promoting a more intentional and mindful approach to their dietary choices.

Enhancement of Emotional Well-Being:

- The ultimate goal of addressing emotional eating is the enhancement of emotional well-being. Through self-awareness, informed decision-making, and the cultivation of healthier coping mechanisms, individuals can navigate emotional challenges more effectively, contributing to a more positive and resilient emotional state.

In summary, addressing emotional eating is a vital component of mindful eating within the context of a low-carb lifestyle. By identifying triggers, fostering self-awareness, and developing healthier coping strategies, individuals can transform their relationship with food, leading to a more balanced and emotionally resilient approach to eating.

The cultivation of healthy coping mechanisms is a crucial aspect of fostering emotional well-being within the context of a low-carb lifestyle. Here are key points elaborating on the significance of developing alternative coping strategies:

Replacing Emotional Eating Patterns:

- The goal of cultivating healthy coping mechanisms is to replace reliance on emotional eating patterns. Instead of turning to food as the primary means of coping with stress or emotions, individuals are encouraged to explore alternative practices that contribute to overall well-being.

Diverse Coping Strategies:

- Healthy coping mechanisms encompass a diverse range of practices tailored to individual preferences. These may include mindfulness meditation, journaling, engaging in physical activity, practicing deep-breathing exercises, or participating in creative outlets. The emphasis is on discovering activities that resonate with the individual and effectively address emotional needs.

Mindfulness Practices:

- Mindfulness techniques, such as meditation and deep-breathing exercises, play a significant role in healthy coping. These practices promote present-moment awareness, helping individuals manage stress and emotions with a calm and focused mindset. Mindfulness also encourages a non-judgmental attitude towards emotions, fostering acceptance and self-compassion.

Journaling for Self-Reflection:
- Journaling provides a constructive outlet for self-reflection and expression of emotions. By putting thoughts and feelings on paper, individuals gain clarity and insight into their emotional landscape. Journaling can be a valuable tool for identifying patterns, tracking triggers, and developing strategies to navigate emotional challenges.

Physical Activity as Stress Relief:

- Engaging in regular physical activity is a powerful way to manage stress and enhance emotional well-being. Exercise releases endorphins, the body's natural mood lifters, and provides an outlet for pent-up energy and tension. Whether through structured workouts, outdoor activities, or simply incorporating movement into daily routines, physical activity contributes to emotional resilience.

Holistic Well-Being:

- The cultivation of healthy coping mechanisms aligns with the broader concept of holistic well-being. It acknowledges that emotional health is interconnected with physical, mental, and social well-being. By addressing emotional needs through diverse coping strategies, individuals contribute to a more comprehensive and balanced approach to their overall health.

Enhanced Emotional Resilience:

- Healthy coping mechanisms contribute to the development of emotional resilience. Instead of relying on external factors like food for emotional regulation, individuals become equipped with a toolkit of strategies to navigate life's challenges. This resilience enhances the capacity to adapt and respond positively to stressors, fostering emotional strength.

Long-Term Sustainable Habits:

- Incorporating healthy coping mechanisms supports the development of sustainable habits. Unlike short-term fixes, these practices can be integrated into daily life for the long term. By establishing a repertoire of coping strategies, individuals create a foundation for lasting emotional well-being and a resilient relationship with food.

Professional Guidance and Support:

- Seeking professional guidance, such as counseling or therapy, can be instrumental in developing healthy coping mechanisms. Trained professionals can provide personalized strategies, guidance, and support tailored to an individual's unique circumstances, facilitating a more effective and targeted approach to emotional well-being.

In summary, developing healthy coping mechanisms is a crucial element of a comprehensive approach to emotional well-being in the context of a low-carb lifestyle. By incorporating a range of coping strategies, individuals can strengthen their emotional resilience, nurture a balanced connection with food, and establish lasting habits that support their overall well-being.

In essence, mindful eating goes beyond the nutritional aspects of a low-carb lifestyle; it encapsulates a holistic approach to nourishing both the body and the soul. Through the integration of mindful eating practices, individuals can foster a profound connection with their meals, listen to the cues of their bodies, and address emotional eating patterns, ultimately contributing to a more mindful and joyous relationship with food.

Navigating Triggers: A Mindful Approach to Dietary Adherence

R ecognizing and avoiding triggers that might lead to deviations from one's dietary plan is a critical aspect of maintaining a successful and sustainable low-carb lifestyle. These triggers, often rooted in emotional or environmental factors, can pose challenges to adhering to dietary goals. One key strategy is to cultivate a heightened awareness of personal triggers, enabling individuals to preemptively navigate situations that may prompt unhealthy eating choices.

Recognizing and understanding triggers for off-plan eating is a fundamental step in developing a mindful and intentional approach to one's relationship with food within a low-carb lifestyle. This process involves a thoughtful exploration of emotional, social, and situational cues that may act as catalysts for veering off the planned dietary path.

Emotional Triggers:

- Emotional triggers encompass a spectrum of feelings, such as stress, anxiety, sadness, or even joy. For some individuals, food becomes a coping mechanism in response to emotional challenges. Identifying these triggers involves introspection to recognize patterns where certain emotions prompt a desire for specific foods.

Social Influences:

- Social gatherings and interactions can significantly impact dietary choices. Peer pressure, cultural norms, and the availability of certain foods in social settings can influence individuals to deviate from their planned low-carb intake. Identifying social triggers involves being mindful of how social dynamics and expectations may affect eating behaviors.

Boredom and Routine:

- Boredom and routine can lead to mindless eating or seeking comfort in familiar foods. Identifying triggers related to boredom involves recognizing instances where the desire to eat arises not out of hunger but as a response to monotony or habit. Breaking the cycle of routine-related triggers is essential for mindful eating.

Environmental Cues:

- Specific environments or surroundings can act as powerful triggers. For example, the workplace, home, or specific areas associated with particular eating habits may influence dietary choices. Identifying environmental triggers requires an awareness of how surroundings can impact food-related decisions and habits.

Situational Challenges:

- Certain situations, such as travel or time constraints, can pose challenges to adhering to a low-carb plan. Recognizing situational triggers involves anticipating potential obstacles and planning ahead to make informed and mindful choices when faced with these challenges.

Self-Reflection and Journaling:

- Engaging in self-reflection and maintaining a food journal can be instrumental in identifying triggers. Recording thoughts, emotions, and circumstances surrounding eating episodes provides a tangible record for analysis. Patterns and trends become apparent, aiding in the identification of recurring triggers.

Proactive Approach:

- The process of identifying triggers empowers individuals to take a proactive stance in managing their response to various cues. By understanding the circumstances that lead to off-plan eating, individuals can implement strategies to navigate these situations more mindfully and make intentional choices aligned with their health goals.

Mindful Decision-Making:

- Armed with insights into triggers, individuals can cultivate mindful decision-making. This involves consciously choosing how to respond to emotional, social, or situational cues, considering the impact on their overall well-being. Mindful decision-making is a key component of building a resilient and intentional approach to food choices.

Identifying triggers for off-plan eating is a thoughtful and introspective process that empowers individuals to navigate their low-carb lifestyle with greater awareness and intention. By recognizing the various cues that influence eating behaviors, individuals can proactively address challenges, make informed choices, and cultivate a sustainable and mindful relationship with food.

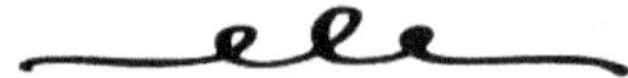

Successfully steering clear of triggers within a low-carb lifestyle demands a comprehensive strategy that integrates mindfulness practices with strategic planning. By combining these elements, individuals can fortify their resilience against potential triggers, fostering a more intentional and successful adherence to their dietary goals.

Mindfulness Techniques:

- *Stress as a Trigger:* For those who identify stress as a trigger, incorporating mindfulness techniques becomes paramount. Practices such as meditation, deep breathing exercises, or mindfulness-based stress reduction can effectively manage stress responses. These techniques empower individuals to navigate challenging situations without resorting to impulsive or emotional eating.

Strategic Planning for Social Events:

- *Navigating Social Influences:* Social events often pose challenges to maintaining a low-carb lifestyle. Strategic planning involves anticipating social triggers and taking proactive steps. This can include communicating dietary preferences to hosts in advance, ensuring there are low-carb alternatives available, or even bringing a dish that aligns with one's dietary choices. This approach minimizes the risk of succumbing to temptations during social gatherings.

Preemptive Measures for Routine Triggers:

- *Breaking the Boredom Cycle:* Recognizing routine or boredom as triggers necessitates preemptive measures. Engaging in activities that break the monotony, incorporating variety into daily routines, or having pre-planned activities to turn to during idle moments can disrupt the cycle of boredom-triggered eating.

Establishing Default Healthy Options:

- *Creating Go-To Choices:* To avoid succumbing to environmental triggers, establishing default healthy options becomes essential. This involves ensuring that convenient and low-carb choices are readily available in common environments, such as the workplace or home. Having go-to snacks or meals that align with dietary goals reduces the likelihood of opting for less healthy alternatives.

Flexibility within Dietary Preferences:

- *Adapting to Social Environments:* Strategic planning also involves recognizing that some social situations may present limited low-carb options. Being flexible within the boundaries of one's dietary preferences allows for adaptability. This might involve making the best choices available in a given situation without compromising overall goals.

Regular Self-Reflection:

- *Monitoring Progress and Adjusting Strategies:* Regular self-reflection is crucial for refining avoidance strategies. Monitoring progress, identifying any new triggers that may emerge, and adjusting strategies accordingly ensure that the approach remains dynamic and aligned with evolving needs.

Mindful Decision-Making in Real Time:

- *Applying Mindfulness in the Moment:* The combination of mindfulness and strategic planning extends to real-time decision-making. In potential triggers, individuals can draw upon mindfulness practices to make conscious and intentional choices that align with their overall health goals.

In conclusion, avoiding triggers within a low-carb lifestyle involves a dynamic interplay of mindfulness and strategic planning. By proactively addressing stress, social situations, routine triggers, and environmental influences, individuals can navigate their dietary journey with resilience and intentionality. This holistic approach not only empowers individuals to avoid common pitfalls but also contributes to the development of sustainable and mindful eating habits.

The creation of a supportive environment stands as a pivotal strategy in the pursuit of trigger avoidance within a low-carb lifestyle. This multifaceted approach involves not only adjusting physical surroundings but also cultivating a positive and understanding social ecosystem. By intertwining these elements, individuals can fortify their commitment to a low-carb journey, minimizing the allure of triggers and reinforcing a steadfast adherence to their dietary goals.

Home Environment:

- *Stocking Low-Carb Options:* The home serves as the primary battleground against triggers. A crucial step involves stocking the pantry and refrigerator with a variety of low-carb options. Having readily accessible, healthy choices ensures that when hunger strikes or cravings emerge, individuals can easily opt for compliant alternatives. This proactive measure minimizes the temptation posed by non-compliant foods.*Minimizing Temptations:* Beyond stocking low-carb options, minimizing the presence of tempting, non-compliant foods is paramount. Clearing the home environment of high-carb snacks, sugary treats, and processed foods reduces the likelihood of impulsive, off-plan eating. This intentional arrangement promotes a visual and physical environment that aligns with the commitment to a low-carb lifestyle.

Social Support System:

- *Positive and Understanding Social Circle:* Surrounding oneself with a supportive social circle is equally crucial. Friends, family, and colleagues who understand and respect one's dietary choices can provide invaluable encouragement. Whether attending social events or navigating daily interactions, having individuals who foster a positive and understanding atmosphere contributes significantly to staying on track during challenging situations.*Communication and Education:* Effective communication about dietary preferences and goals with those in one's social circle is foundational. Educating others about the principles of a low-carb lifestyle helps establish a shared understanding. This communication can also preemptively address potential challenges in social settings, allowing for a collaborative effort in creating an environment that supports rather than hinders dietary goals.

Cultivating a Positive Atmosphere:

- *Encouragement and Positivity:* The creation of a supportive environment extends beyond physical surroundings to the emotional atmosphere. Encouragement and positivity from those around can be a powerful motivator. Celebrating achievements, no matter how small, and offering support during challenging times contribute to a positive atmosphere that reinforces the commitment to a low-carb lifestyle.*Collaborative Meal Planning:* In social settings, collaborative meal planning can be a unifying activity. Whether with family or friends, involving others in the planning and preparation of low-carb meals fosters a sense of shared commitment. This collaborative approach not only strengthens relationships but also ensures that social gatherings align with dietary goals.

Flexible and Inclusive Approach:

- *Accommodating Different Preferences:* A supportive environment acknowledges and accommodates diverse dietary preferences. This inclusivity allows individuals to navigate social situations without feeling isolated or pressured to deviate from their chosen path. A flexible and understanding approach from those in one's social circle contributes to a harmonious coexistence of varied dietary choices.

Education and Awareness:

- *Disseminating Information:* Education plays a crucial role in creating a supportive environment. Disseminating accurate information about the benefits and principles of a low-carb lifestyle helps dispel misconceptions. This shared knowledge fosters an environment where individuals can make informed choices and offer constructive support based on a clear understanding of the underlying principles.

By curating a home environment conducive to low-carb choices and cultivating a positive, understanding social circle, individuals create a foundation that empowers them to navigate challenges with resilience. This holistic approach not only safeguards against triggers but also cultivates an atmosphere that nurtures a sustained commitment to a low-carb lifestyle.

Additionally, establishing healthy coping mechanisms is pivotal in navigating triggers successfully. Rather than turning to food for emotional relief, individuals can explore alternative outlets like engaging in physical activity, practicing mindfulness, or seeking support from friends and family. Building a repertoire of positive coping strategies reinforces resilience against triggers and empowers individuals to make mindful choices aligned with their dietary goals.

In conclusion, recognizing and avoiding triggers that may lead to dietary deviations is a dynamic process rooted in self-awareness and proactive planning. By acknowledging personal triggers, implementing strategies for avoidance, and cultivating healthy coping mechanisms, individuals on a low-carb journey can fortify their commitment to a balanced and sustainable dietary lifestyle. This mindful approach not only promotes dietary adherence but also fosters a positive and empowered relationship with food.

Socializing and Dining Out: Crafting a Low-Carb Social Experience

Embarking on a low-carb lifestyle doesn't mean bidding farewell to socializing and dining out; rather, it involves navigating these situations with mindfulness and informed choices. A key aspect of successfully managing social situations is effective communication of dietary preferences. Whether attending gatherings or dining with friends, openly communicating one's dietary choices ensures a supportive and understanding environment. This may involve informing hosts in advance or engaging in open dialogue with friends about the low-carb journey, fostering a collaborative approach to social events.

Mastering the art of making informed choices at restaurants is a pivotal skill within the low-carb toolkit, enabling individuals to maintain their dietary goals while enjoying dining out. As the culinary landscape evolves, many eateries now recognize and cater to diverse dietary preferences, providing a spectrum of options. The following guidelines offer insights into navigating restaurant menus strategically, empowering individuals to make choices that align with the principles of a low-carb lifestyle:

- Focus on Nutrient-Dense Options:

  - *Lean Proteins:* Prioritize dishes featuring lean proteins such as poultry, fish, lean cuts of meat, and plant-based protein sources. Grilled or roasted preparations are often excellent choices, offering flavorful protein without added carbohydrates.

- *Healthy Fats:* Seek out dishes incorporating healthy fats, such as those from avocados, nuts, seeds, and olive oil. These fats not only enhance the satiety of the meal but also align with the macronutrient profile of a balanced low-carb diet.

- Embrace Non-Starchy Vegetables:

  - *Vegetable-Centric Dishes:* Opt for dishes where non-starchy vegetables take center stage. Salads with protein toppings, vegetable stir-fries, or grilled vegetable platters provide a satisfying and low-carb foundation.

  - *Varied Color Palette:* Choose a variety of colorful vegetables to ensure a diverse range of nutrients. Incorporating leafy greens, cruciferous vegetables, and vibrant bell peppers adds both nutritional value and visual appeal to the meal.

- Strategic Carbohydrate Substitutions:

  - *Cauliflower as a Substitute:* Explore menu options that allow for substitutions, particularly when it comes to high-carb sides. Cauliflower rice, for instance, can replace traditional rice, offering a low-carb alternative that complements various dishes.

  - *Zucchini Noodles:* In pasta-based dishes, inquire about the possibility of substituting regular noodles with zucchini noodles. This swap not only reduces carb content but introduces an additional serving of vegetables.

- Grilled and Roasted Preparations:

- *Grilled Proteins:* Opting for grilled or roasted proteins is a low-carb strategy that avoids breading or excessive added carbohydrates. Grilled chicken, fish, or lean cuts of meat are flavorful choices that align with the principles of a low-carb lifestyle.

- *Roasted Vegetables:* Choose sides featuring roasted vegetables, as roasting enhances their natural flavors without relying on high-carb preparations. This method of cooking complements the low-carb approach by preserving the integrity of ingredients.

- **Customize to Your Preference:**

  - *Communication with Servers:* Don't hesitate to communicate dietary preferences with restaurant staff. Many establishments are accommodating and willing to tailor dishes to meet specific requirements. Clear communication ensures that the meal is prepared in a way that aligns with the low-carb goals.

- **Portion Control:**

  - *Mindful Portions:* Be mindful of portion sizes, as restaurant servings can sometimes be larger than necessary. Consider sharing dishes or opting for appetizer portions to manage calorie and carbohydrate intake effectively.

- **Beverage Choices:**

  - *Hydration:* Choose water or other low-carb beverages to stay hydrated without adding unnecessary sugars. Avoid sugary sodas or high-calorie drinks that can contribute to excess carbohydrate intake.

By adopting these strategies, individuals can approach restaurant dining with confidence, knowing they have the tools to make informed choices that align with their low-carb lifestyle. This skill not only enhances the dining experience but also empowers individuals to enjoy a variety of culinary offerings while staying true to their dietary goals.

Successfully navigating social situations and dining out is a skill that complements a low-carb lifestyle, providing individuals with the flexibility to enjoy diverse culinary experiences while adhering to their dietary goals. Making informed and health-conscious choices in these scenarios involves strategic decision-making and an understanding of which options align with low-carb principles. Here are key considerations for identifying healthy low-carb options in social and dining-out settings:

- Grilled Proteins:

  - *Lean Meat and Fish:* Opt for dishes featuring grilled or broiled lean proteins, such as chicken, turkey, fish, or lean cuts of beef. Grilled preparations often enhance the natural flavors of the protein without the need for high-carb coatings.

- Salads with Vinaigrette Dressing:

  - *Vegetable-Centric Salads:* Explore salads that showcase a variety of non-starchy vegetables, accompanied by a vinaigrette dressing. This combination provides a refreshing and low-carb option, allowing individuals to enjoy a nutrient-dense meal.

- Vegetable-Centric Appetizers:

  - *Diverse Culinary Offerings:* Scan the appetizer section for options that emphasize vegetables and lean proteins. Vegetable-centric appetizers, such as grilled asparagus, stuffed mushrooms, or skewers with colorful veggies, offer a flavorful start to the meal without excessive carbohydrates.

- Cuisine Diversity:

  - *Mediterranean Options:* Embrace the diversity of cuisines, as various culinary traditions offer flavorful low-carb choices. Mediterranean cuisine, for example, often features dishes rich in olive oil, vegetables, and lean proteins, making it a suitable option for those following a low-carb lifestyle.

  - *Stir-Fried Tofu with Vegetables:* In Asian cuisine, look for stir-fried tofu with a variety of vegetables. This dish provides a satisfying and low-carb alternative, showcasing the versatility of tofu as a protein source.

- Low-Carb Sides and Modifications:

  - *Cauliflower Rice Substitutions:* Check if the restaurant offers low-carb side options or allows for modifications. Swapping traditional rice for cauliflower rice is a popular substitution that aligns with a low-carb approach.

- Mindful Exploration of Menus:

  - *Scan for Keywords:* When perusing menus, pay attention to keywords that indicate healthier and lower-carb options, such as "grilled," "roasted," or "vegetable-centric." These descriptors guide individuals toward choices that align with their dietary preferences.

- Communication with Servers:

  - *Clarify Dietary Preferences:* Communicate dietary preferences with servers, especially if specific modifications or substitutions are desired. Most restaurants are accommodating and can provide valuable insights into the preparation of dishes to meet individual needs.

- Beverage Choices:

  - *Opt for Low-Carb Beverages:* Choose beverages that align with low-carb principles, such as water, unsweetened tea, or sparkling water. This ensures hydration without the addition of unnecessary sugars.

By adopting these strategies, individuals can approach social dining with confidence, knowing that they can make enjoyable and health-conscious choices in a variety of culinary settings. This skill not only enhances the social experience but also reinforces the idea that a low-carb lifestyle is adaptable and sustainable in diverse social and dining contexts.

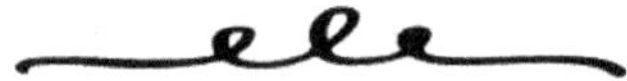

In essence, socializing and dining out can seamlessly integrate with a low-carb lifestyle through effective communication, informed choices, and a keen eye for healthy options. By approaching social situations with confidence, individuals can savor flavorful meals while staying true to their dietary preferences. This balanced approach not only enhances the enjoyment of social experiences but also reinforces the sustainability of a low-carb lifestyle in diverse and dynamic social settings.

Overcoming Challenges and Plateaus: Sustaining Momentum on the Low-Carb Journey

As individuals embark on the journey of a low-carb lifestyle, they inevitably encounter challenges and plateaus that may test their resolve. Addressing these hurdles with resilience and strategic approaches is fundamental to achieving long-term success in maintaining a low-carb diet.

Common Challenges on a Low-Carb Diet

Navigating cravings and resisting the temptation of carb-rich foods constitutes a noteworthy aspect of maintaining a low-carb lifestyle. The allure of comfort foods and sugary treats can be particularly pronounced, often peaking during stressful periods or emotional moments. Effectively managing these cravings requires a nuanced approach that integrates mindful eating practices.

- Mindful eating involves developing a heightened awareness of the eating experience. It begins with recognizing the subtle but crucial distinction between emotional and physical hunger. Identifying whether the desire to eat stems from genuine physiological needs or emotional triggers lays the foundation for making conscious and informed choices.

- During moments of craving, it becomes essential to pause and assess the nature of the hunger. Is it driven by an actual need for sustenance, or is it a response to stress, boredom, or other emotional factors? This reflective pause provides an opportunity to address the root cause of the craving.

- Finding satisfying low-carb alternatives is a key strategy in managing cravings. Rather than succumbing to the allure of high-carb comfort foods, individuals can explore and incorporate alternatives that align with their dietary goals. This might involve having a selection of nutrient-dense snacks readily available, such as nuts, seeds, or low-carb vegetables, to provide a sense of satiety without compromising the commitment to a low-carb lifestyle.

- Moreover, mindful eating practices encourage individuals to savor and appreciate the flavors and textures of the foods they choose. By consciously engaging with the eating process, individuals can derive greater satisfaction from their meals, diminishing the allure of indulging in carb-heavy treats simply out of habit or impulse.

- The effective management of cravings within a low-carb lifestyle revolves around the cultivation of self-awareness and the intentional selection of satisfying, low-carb alternatives. This approach not only supports adherence to dietary goals but also fosters a positive and mindful relationship with food, empowering individuals to make choices that contribute to their overall well-being.

Dealing with Plateaus

- Encountering plateaus in the pursuit of health goals, where progress appears to stall, is a common and natural occurrence. Recognizing that plateaus are an inherent part of any health journey is fundamental to maintaining a resilient and positive mindset.

- Plateaus may signify that the body has adapted to current dietary and exercise routines, prompting the need for strategic adjustments. Rather than viewing plateaus as setbacks, they can be reframed as opportunities for reassessment and refinement of one's approach.

- To overcome plateaus, individuals can consider various adjustments. Reassessing portion sizes is one avenue, ensuring that caloric intake aligns with the body's current needs and metabolic state. Diversifying exercise routines is another strategy, as the body can adapt to repetitive workouts, leading to diminished returns. Introducing new forms of physical activity or modifying the intensity and duration of existing routines can stimulate progress.

- Experimenting with different low-carb food choices is also a valuable tactic. While adhering to a low-carb lifestyle, the variety of food options within this framework is extensive. Trying new recipes, incorporating a broader range of vegetables, or exploring different sources of lean proteins and healthy fats can introduce novel elements to the diet, potentially breaking through the plateau.

- Maintaining patience and persistence during plateaus is essential. Rather than becoming disheartened, individuals can view plateaus as opportunities for learning more about their bodies and refining their strategies for long-term success. Seeking guidance from healthcare professionals or nutrition experts can provide valuable insights tailored to individual needs, assisting in the formulation of a customized approach to navigate plateaus and continue progressing toward health and wellness goals.

Strategies for Long-Term Success

- In the realm of a low-carb lifestyle, the foundation of long-term success lies in the art of setting realistic and achievable goals. These goals serve as a compass, guiding individuals on their journey toward improved health and well-being. The significance of these objectives extends beyond mere milestones; they are the pillars of sustainable change.

- Realistic goals are essential in preventing the pitfalls of frustration and deprivation. By acknowledging individual starting points, considering personal preferences, and factoring in the demands of daily life, individuals can craft goals that are challenging yet attainable. This balanced approach fosters a positive mindset, creating a pathway where progress can be celebrated, and setbacks can be navigated with resilience.

- The key to success within a low-carb lifestyle is gradual change. Rapid transformations may yield short-term results, but the sustainability of these changes is often compromised. Gradual adjustments, on the other hand, allow for the integration of new habits into existing routines. This methodical approach ensures that dietary and lifestyle changes become ingrained in daily life, increasing the likelihood of long-term adherence and success.

- Setting realistic goals involves a nuanced understanding of individual needs, preferences, and potential challenges. It requires a thoughtful assessment of current habits and a vision for the desired future. Whether the goal is weight management, improved metabolic health, or enhanced well-being, each step forward should be tailored to the individual, creating a trajectory that aligns with their unique journey towards lasting health.

Building a Support System:

- The power of a support system cannot be overstated. Building connections with like-minded individuals, whether friends, family, or online communities, creates a network of encouragement and shared experiences. Having a support system provides emotional reinforcement during challenging moments, offers guidance through plateaus, and celebrates achievements, fostering a sense of camaraderie and motivation.

In conclusion, overcoming challenges and plateaus on a low-carb journey is a dynamic process that demands adaptability and perseverance. By addressing common challenges like cravings and plateaus with mindful strategies, individuals can navigate these obstacles with resilience. Equally important is the cultivation of a supportive environment through realistic goal-setting and the establishment of a robust support system. In tandem, these strategies contribute to sustained momentum, ensuring that the low-carb lifestyle becomes a rewarding and enduring facet of one's health and well-being.

Tracking Progress and Adjusting Goals: The Dynamic Path to Success

Monitoring progress and making necessary adjustments are integral elements of a successful low-carb journey, ensuring that individuals stay attuned to their goals and can adapt their strategies as needed. The process involves a dual focus on tracking various aspects of the journey and being open to making informed adjustments.

Within the realm of a low-carb lifestyle, the meticulous tracking of food intake stands as a fundamental practice for monitoring progress and promoting success. This meticulous record-keeping extends beyond merely quantifying macronutrients; it involves a comprehensive documentation of the types and quality of foods consumed.

Keeping a meticulous record of food intake is more than a routine task; it serves as a potent instrument for individuals on their journey toward a healthier lifestyle. This practice allows for a comprehensive exploration of dietary patterns, offering valuable insights into individual habits, preferences, and areas ripe for improvement. Through this detailed record-keeping, individuals can cultivate heightened awareness, providing a nuanced understanding of their nutritional choices.

This heightened awareness is a key element in the evaluation of dietary practices, enabling individuals to make precise assessments of their nutritional journey. The recorded information becomes a mirror, reflecting not only the strengths in one's dietary approach but also shedding light on aspects that may benefit from adjustment. In essence, the act of tracking food intake is a strategic and informed endeavor, empowering individuals to navigate their nutritional landscape with a tailored and insightful perspective.

This approach to tracking plays a crucial role in maintaining adherence to low-carb principles. It acts as a guiding compass, allowing individuals to gauge their progress, stay accountable to their health goals, and make informed choices aligned with the principles of their low-carb lifestyle. The ability to observe trends in food consumption empowers individuals to navigate challenges, make strategic adjustments, and celebrate successes along their journey.

Furthermore, the record-keeping process becomes a personalized journey of self-discovery, shedding light on the intricate relationship between food choices and individual well-being. It fosters a sense of responsibility and ownership over one's health, laying the foundation for a sustainable and informed low-carb lifestyle. Ultimately, meticulous tracking emerges as a cornerstone in the pursuit of health, offering a roadmap for continuous improvement and ensuring that the principles of the low-carb lifestyle are seamlessly integrated into daily life.

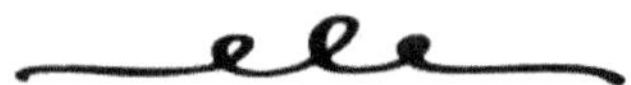

Here are some key points you can include in your daily journal:
- Date:

- Today's Goal:

- Daily Carb Limit in Grams:

- Breakfast

  ○ Type and quantity of food consumed

- Total carb intake for breakfast

- Lunch

  - Food choices including portions

  - Monitor Carb intake and correct as needed

- Snacks

  - Track any snacks consumed

  - Note the carb content aligns with daily goals

- Dinner

  - List dinner options and ingredients

  - Sum up the carb count for the evening meal

- Daily water intake

  - Aim for at least 8 glass (64 ozs. per day)

- Physical Activity

  - Note any exercise or physical activity undertaken

- How do you feel today?

- Rate your energy levels (1-10)

- Record any noticeable changes in mood or well-being

- Challenges encountered:

  - Identify any obstacles faced during the day

  - Brainstorm solutions or adjustments for the future

- Victories Celebrated!

  ○ Acknowledge achievements and milestones reached

- Reflections

- What went well today?

- What could be improved?

- What strategies can be implemented for better success tomorrow?

- Notes:

Additional Tips:

- Meal Planning: Prepare meals and snacks in advance to stay on track.

- Variety Matters: Explore diverse low-carb food options to avoid monotony.

- Read Labels: Scrutinize nutritional labels for accurate carb information.

- Support System: Connect with others on a similar journey for motivation and advice.

Remember, progress is a journey, not a destination. Stay committed, stay positive, and let this journal be your companion in achieving your low-carb lifestyle goals!

Similarly, tracking physical activity is crucial for a comprehensive understanding of progress. Whether through fitness apps, journals, or wearable devices, tracking physical activity allows individuals to gauge their efforts, celebrate achievements, and identify areas where adjustments may be necessary. This dual approach to tracking fosters a holistic perspective on health and well-being.

Moving on to making adjustments, regular and periodic assessments are key to making informed adjustments. These assessments involve a comprehensive review of both dietary and physical activity logs. Evaluating progress against initial goals, considering overall well-being, and reflecting on challenges and successes form the foundation of these assessments. Periodic reassessments empower individuals to recalibrate their goals, modify strategies, and embrace a dynamic approach to their low-carb journey.

In essence, tracking progress and adjusting goals are dynamic processes that fortify the adaptability and sustainability of a low-carb lifestyle. Through meticulous monitoring of food intake and physical activity, individuals gain a nuanced understanding of their journey. This awareness, coupled with periodic assessments, empowers individuals to make informed adjustments, ensuring that their goals remain realistic, attainable, and aligned with the evolving nature of their health and wellness objectives.

Adapting to Changing Needs: The Flexible Framework of a Low-Carb Lifestyle

E mbracing a low-carb diet is not a static endeavor; it's a dynamic journey that requires adaptability to changing needs over time. Life is inherently dynamic, marked by shifting priorities, evolving schedules, and varying health requirements. Navigating these changes while maintaining a low-carb lifestyle involves cultivating a flexible mindset and adopting strategies that align with one's current needs.

Understanding Changing Needs:

Navigating the ebb and flow of life involves a profound understanding of changing needs, particularly when it comes to the dynamic nature of individual circumstances. Life is marked by transitions – shifts in work schedules, evolving family dynamics, and changes in health status, all of which can significantly influence dietary preferences and requirements.

The key to effectively adapting to changing needs begins with a keen awareness of these shifts. By recognizing the evolving landscape of one's life, individuals can proactively assess and understand the impact on their low-carb lifestyle. This recognition serves as the compass, guiding them to tailor their approach in alignment with their current needs. Whether it's adjusting meal plans, reconsidering food choices, or modifying eating schedules, the ability to adapt to changing needs is a fundamental skill in sustaining a well-rounded and flexible low-carb lifestyle.

Flexible Meal Planning:

In the realm of a low-carb lifestyle, the importance of meal planning cannot be overstated; it serves as a cornerstone for success. However, recognizing the dynamic nature of life, where schedules evolve, priorities shift, and energy demands fluctuate, emphasizes the need for flexible meal planning.

Flexible meal planning is a strategic approach that acknowledges the ever-changing circumstances individuals may encounter. This adaptability ensures that meal plans remain aligned with the fundamental principles of a low-carb lifestyle while catering to specific needs. Whether facing time constraints or seeking to boost energy levels, flexible meal planning allows for the inclusion of diverse, nutrient-dense options. It provides the necessary agility to navigate through various scenarios without compromising the commitment to a low-carb way of eating.

The beauty of flexible meal planning lies in its capacity to accommodate shifts in dietary requirements seamlessly. By embracing this adaptability, individuals can create sustainable and enjoyable meal plans that not only contribute to their health goals but also effortlessly integrate into the rhythm of their evolving lifestyles.

Smart Substitutions:

The concept of adaptability within a low-carb lifestyle is synonymous with making intelligent substitutions that cater to evolving needs. This strategic approach becomes particularly relevant during periods of increased activity or heightened stress levels, where individuals may require quick and convenient sources of energy.

In such situations, opting for low-carb snacks that are both efficient and satisfying, such as nuts or cheese, becomes a practical choice. These alternatives not only align with the low-carb principles but also provide the necessary fuel to meet heightened energy demands. The ability to make these smart substitutions enables individuals to seamlessly integrate their dietary choices with the demands of their dynamic lifestyles.

Furthermore, the exploration of new low-carb recipes and the incorporation of seasonal produce contribute to the adaptability of the dietary approach. This not only adds variety to the menu but also addresses changing taste preferences. Embracing a diverse range of foods ensures that individuals can enjoy the flexibility inherent in a low-carb lifestyle without compromising nutritional quality, thereby enhancing the overall sustainability and satisfaction of their dietary choices.

Periodic Reevaluation:

Regular reassessment of dietary goals and health needs stands as a fundamental and proactive aspect of adapting to change within a low-carb lifestyle. The practice of periodic evaluations serves multiple purposes, offering individuals a structured framework to reflect on their progress, refine their goals, and make informed adjustments to their dietary approaches.

These assessments provide a valuable opportunity for individuals to gauge the effectiveness of their current low-carb strategy, taking into account various factors such as weight management, energy levels, and overall well-being. By scrutinizing the outcomes against initially set goals, individuals can identify areas of success and pinpoint aspects that might require modification.

This reflective process also allows for the adjustment of goals to align with evolving health needs or changing circumstances. It acknowledges that personal priorities, health conditions, or lifestyle factors may shift over time, necessitating modifications to dietary preferences or nutritional requirements. The ability to fine-tune dietary approaches based on these assessments ensures that the low-carb lifestyle remains not only effective but also supportive and sustainable.

In essence, regular reassessment serves as a proactive measure, empowering individuals to navigate their health journey with flexibility and responsiveness. By fostering a continuous feedback loop, individuals can optimize their approach to low-carb living, ensuring its enduring relevance and effectiveness in meeting their evolving health and wellness objectives.

Seeking Professional Guidance:

In times of significant changes, seeking guidance from healthcare professionals or nutritionists is a prudent and proactive step within the realm of a low-carb lifestyle. These experts, armed with extensive knowledge and expertise, play a crucial role in providing personalized advice tailored to an individual's unique health circumstances and dietary needs.

Healthcare professionals possess the training and insights necessary to interpret how specific changes, be they related to health conditions, lifestyle modifications, or other factors, may impact nutritional requirements. By consulting with these experts, individuals can gain a deeper understanding of how to navigate the complexities of their evolving health landscape while staying committed to the principles of a low-carb framework.

Nutritionists, in particular, specialize in crafting dietary plans that align with individual health goals and needs. They can offer strategic advice on adapting low-carb approaches to accommodate changing circumstances, ensuring that nutritional adequacy is maintained even in the face of significant life transitions.

Moreover, healthcare professionals and nutritionists serve as valuable sources of support, providing evidence-based recommendations that promote overall well-being. Their guidance extends beyond the immediate challenges of adapting to change, contributing to a sustained and healthful low-carb lifestyle that evolves in tandem with an individual's health journey.

Seeking guidance from healthcare professionals or nutritionists underscores a commitment to maintaining a holistic and well-informed approach to health, where expert advice complements personal efforts, fostering a resilient and adaptable low-carb lifestyle.

In conclusion, adapting to changing needs while maintaining a low-carb diet is a testament to the flexibility inherent in a well-structured dietary approach. By understanding individual circumstances, embracing flexible meal planning, making smart substitutions, and periodically reevaluating goals, individuals can navigate life's transitions while staying committed to the health-enhancing benefits of a low-carb lifestyle.

Conclusion: Nurturing Your Journey Towards Wellness

Recap of Key Concepts:

In our exploration of the realms of a healthy low-carb lifestyle, we've journeyed through foundational principles, mindful practices, and adaptive strategies. Key concepts such as mindful eating, balanced nutrition, and the symbiotic relationship between physical activity and dietary choices have emerged as cornerstones. Recognizing and addressing challenges, tracking progress, and adapting to changing needs form a dynamic framework that fosters sustained well-being.

Encouragement for Sustaining a Healthy Low-Carb Lifestyle:

As we conclude this journey, it's essential to emphasize that embracing a healthy low-carb lifestyle is not a destination but a continuous path toward well-being. The journey is marked by successes, challenges, and periods of growth. Your commitment to mindful choices, balanced nutrition, and an active lifestyle is a testament to your dedication to personal health.

Celebrate your victories, no matter how small, and recognize that each step contributes to the tapestry of your well-being.

Remember that setbacks are not failures but opportunities to learn and readjust. The sustainable nature of a low-carb lifestyle lies in its adaptability to your evolving needs. Your body is a dynamic entity, and your approach to health should reflect that dynamism. Continue to listen to your body, make informed choices, and nurture a positive relationship with food and physical activity.

Additional Resources for Continued Support:

For ongoing support in your low-carb journey, a wealth of resources is available to you. From reputable websites and books to online communities and nutrition experts, these resources offer a rich tapestry of knowledge, guidance, and community support. Consider exploring cookbooks with creative low-carb recipes, engaging in forums to share experiences and insights, and consulting with healthcare professionals or registered dietitians for personalized advice.

Here are a few recommended resources to continue your journey:

- On the Web: *LowCarbPractitioners.com*

- In Print: The South Beach Diet: The Delicious, Doctor-Designed, Foolproof Plan for Fast and Healthy Weight Loss by Dr. Arthur Agatston

- Dr. Atkins' Diet Revolution by Dr. Robert Atkins

As you progress on your health journey, it's essential to recognize that maintaining well-being is a lifelong commitment. The choices you make today are instrumental in establishing the groundwork for a vibrant and fulfilling future. Your steadfast dedication to a healthy low-carb lifestyle represents a valuable gift to yourself—a strategic investment in the longevity and overall well-being that will accompany you throughout your life's journey.

The commitment to a low-carb lifestyle transcends mere dietary choices; it is a holistic pledge to prioritize your health and vitality. By embracing this approach, you are not only making positive changes in the present but also cultivating habits that contribute to sustained well-being in the years to come.

This dedication is akin to an investment—a conscious and deliberate effort to enhance your quality of life. The benefits of a healthy low-carb lifestyle extend beyond the immediate, impacting your energy levels, cognitive function, and overall resilience. Each wholesome choice contributes to the cumulative wealth of your health, creating a robust foundation for a future marked by optimal physical and mental well-being.

Remember that health is a dynamic and evolving journey, and your commitment to a low-carb lifestyle positions you as an active participant in your wellness. By making informed choices today, you are proactively shaping the narrative of your health and setting the stage for a future characterized by vitality, longevity, and the fulfillment of your well-being goals.

As we bring this journey to a close, it's important to note that this is not a farewell but an invitation—an invitation to persist in your exploration of health and wellness. May your path ahead be illuminated with boundless energy, profound joy, and the deep satisfaction that comes from nurturing both your body and mind through the enriching principles of a healthy low-carb lifestyle.

As you navigate this ongoing adventure, may you find inspiration in the positive changes you've embraced and the transformative power of your choices. Here's to the continued cultivation of your well-being—a toast to a future filled with vitality, happiness, and the enduring rewards of your commitment to a life well-lived.

Cheers to your sustained well-being, and may each step forward bring you closer to the vibrant and fulfilling life you deserve!

Appendix: Additional Recipes!

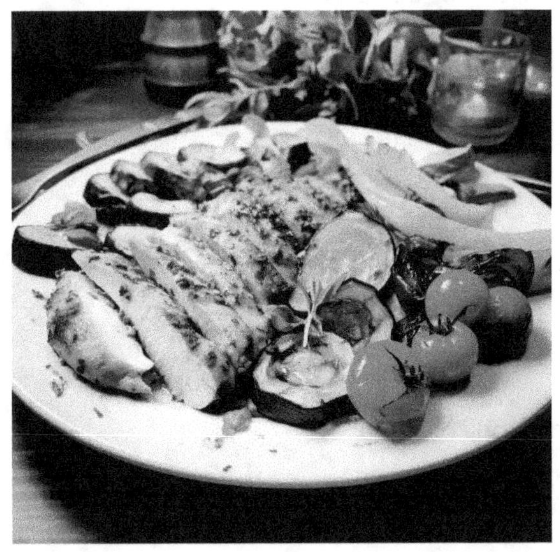

Grilled Lemon Herb Chicken with Roasted Vegetables

Ingredients:

- 2 boneless, skinless chicken breasts

- 1 lemon (zested and juiced)

- 2 tablespoons olive oil

- 2 cloves garlic (minced)

- 1 teaspoon dried oregano

- 1 teaspoon dried thyme

- Salt and black pepper to taste

For the Roasted Vegetables:

- 1 zucchini, sliced

- 1 red bell pepper, sliced

- 1 yellow bell pepper, sliced

- 1 cup cherry tomatoes

- 1 red onion, sliced

- 2 tablespoons olive oil

- Salt and black pepper to taste

- Fresh herbs for garnish (optional)

Instructions:

1. Marinate the Chicken:

- In a bowl, combine lemon zest, lemon juice, olive oil, minced garlic, dried oregano, dried thyme, salt, and black pepper.

- Place the chicken breasts in a resealable plastic bag and pour half of the marinade over them. Seal the bag and refrigerate for at least 30 minutes (or longer for better flavor).

2. Prepare the Vegetables:

- Preheat your oven to 400°F (200°C).

- In a large baking dish, toss the sliced zucchini, bell peppers, cherry tomatoes, and red onion with olive oil, salt, and black pepper.

3. Roast the Vegetables:

- Roast the vegetables in the preheated oven for about 20-25 minutes or until they are tender and slightly caramelized. Stir occasionally for even cooking.

4. Grill the Chicken:

- Preheat a grill or grill pan over medium-high heat.

- Grill the marinated chicken breasts for 6-8 minutes per side or until fully cooked. The internal temperature should reach 165°F (74°C).

5. Serve:

- Place the grilled chicken on a plate alongside the roasted vegetables.

- Garnish with fresh herbs if desired.

This flavorful and wholesome low-carb dinner is rich in protein and fiber while keeping the carb content in check. Feel free to customize the vegetables or herbs to suit your taste preferences. Enjoy your delicious and nutritious meal!

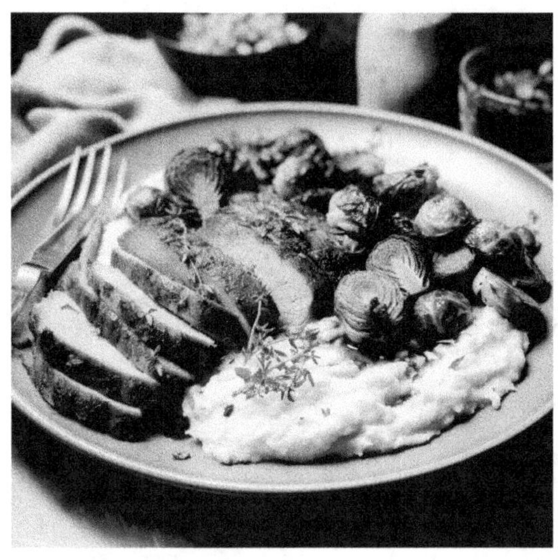

Herb-Roasted Pork Tenderloin with Cauliflower Mash and Roasted Brussels Sprouts

Ingredients:

For the Pork:

- 2 pork tenderloins (about 1 pound each)

- 2 tablespoons olive oil

- 2 cloves garlic (minced)

- 1 teaspoon dried rosemary

- 1 teaspoon dried thyme

- Salt and black pepper to taste

For the Cauliflower Mash:

- 1 large head of cauliflower, cut into florets

- 2 tablespoons unsalted butter

- 1/4 cup heavy cream

- Salt and black pepper to taste

For the Roasted Brussels Sprouts:
- 1 pound Brussels sprouts, trimmed and halved

- 2 tablespoons olive oil

- Salt and black pepper to taste

Instructions:

1. Prepare the Pork:
   - Preheat your oven to 400°F (200°C).

   - In a small bowl, mix olive oil, minced garlic, dried rosemary, dried thyme, salt, and black pepper.

   - Rub the pork tenderloins with the herb mixture, ensuring they are well coated.

2. Roast the Pork:
   - Place the pork tenderloins on a baking sheet lined with parchment paper.

   - Roast in the preheated oven for 20-25 minutes or until the internal temperature reaches 145°F (63°C).

   - Allow the pork to rest for a few minutes before slicing.

3. Prepare the Cauliflower Mash:

- Steam or boil the cauliflower florets until tender.

- Drain the cauliflower and transfer it to a food processor.

- Add butter, heavy cream, salt, and black pepper. Blend until smooth and creamy.

4. Roast the Brussels Sprouts:
   - Toss the halved Brussels sprouts with olive oil, salt, and black pepper.

   - Roast in the oven for 20-25 minutes or until they are golden brown and crispy on the edges.

5. Serve:
   - Slice the herb-roasted pork tenderloin and serve it alongside a generous scoop of cauliflower mash and roasted Brussels sprouts.

This low-carb dinner is not only delicious but also packed with protein and healthy fats. It's a well-balanced meal that will leave you satisfied without compromising your low-carb lifestyle. Enjoy your flavorful and nutritious dinner!

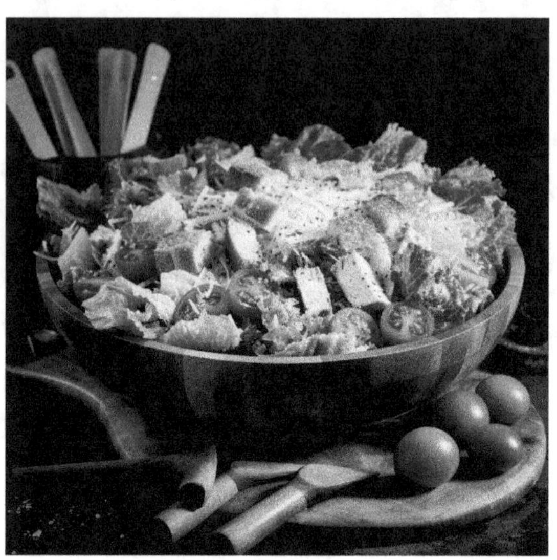

Chicken Caesar Salad and Vegetable Soup

Ingredients:

For the Salad:
- 2 boneless, skinless chicken breasts

- Salt and black pepper to taste

- 1 tablespoon olive oil

- Romaine lettuce, washed and chopped

- Cherry tomatoes, halved

- Parmesan cheese, shaved

For the Caesar Dressing:
- 1/2 cup mayonnaise

- 2 tablespoons grated Parmesan cheese

- 2 teaspoons Dijon mustard

- 1 clove garlic, minced

- 1 tablespoon lemon juice

- Salt and black pepper to taste

For the Soup:
- 4 cups chicken broth (homemade or low-sodium store-bought)

- 1 cup cauliflower florets

- 1 cup broccoli florets

- 1 medium carrot, sliced

- 2 cloves garlic, minced

- 1 teaspoon dried thyme

- Salt and black pepper to taste

- Chopped fresh parsley for garnish

Instructions:

For the Chicken Caesar Salad:

1. Cook the Chicken:
- Season the chicken breasts with salt and black pepper.

- In a skillet, heat olive oil over medium-high heat.

- Cook the chicken breasts for 6-7 minutes per side or until cooked through.

- Let them rest for a few minutes, then slice into strips.

2. Prepare the Caesar Dressing:
   - In a small bowl, whisk together mayonnaise, grated Parmesan cheese, Dijon mustard, minced garlic, lemon juice, salt, and black pepper.

3. Assemble the Salad:
   - In a large bowl, combine chopped romaine lettuce, cherry tomatoes, and sliced chicken.

   - Drizzle the Caesar dressing over the salad and toss until well coated.

   - Top with shaved Parmesan cheese.

For the Low-Carb Soup:

1. Cook the Vegetables:

- In a pot, combine chicken broth, cauliflower, broccoli, carrot, minced garlic, dried thyme, salt, and black pepper.

- Bring to a boil, then reduce the heat and simmer until the vegetables are tender.

2. Blend the Soup:

- Use an immersion blender to blend the soup until smooth. Alternatively, transfer the soup to a blender in batches and blend until smooth.

3. Serve:

Ladle the soup into bowls, garnish with chopped fresh parsley, and serve alongside the Chicken Caesar Salad.

This low-carb Chicken Caesar Salad paired with vegetable soup makes for a satisfying and nutritious lunch. It's a perfect balance of protein, healthy fats, and veggies while keeping the carb count low. Enjoy your delicious and wholesome meal!

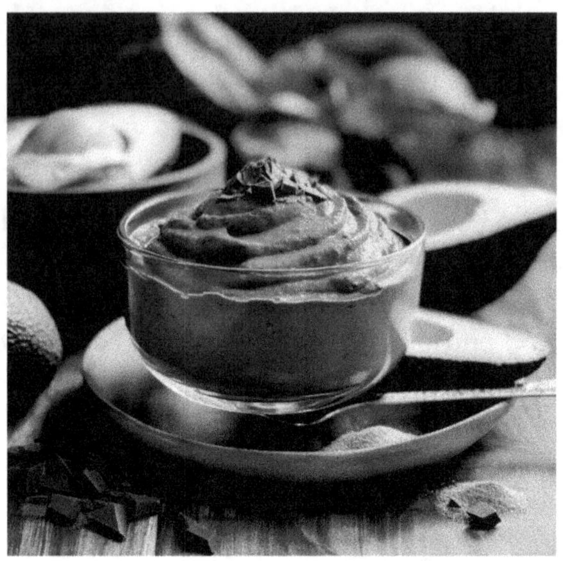

Low-Carb Chocolate Avocado Mousse:

Ingredients:

- 2 ripe avocados

- 1/4 cup unsweetened cocoa powder

- 1/4 cup almond milk (unsweetened)

- 1/4 cup low-carb sweetener (like Erythritol or Stevia), adjust to taste

- 1 teaspoon vanilla extract

- A pinch of salt

- Optional toppings: whipped cream, berries, or chopped nuts

Instructions:

- Prepare the Avocados:

  - Cut the avocados in half, remove the pits, and scoop the flesh into a blender or food processor.

- Blend Ingredients:

  - Add cocoa powder, almond milk, low-carb sweetener, vanilla extract, and a pinch of salt to the blender or food processor.

- Blend Until Smooth:

  - Blend the ingredients until smooth and creamy. Scrape down the sides as needed to ensure everything is well incorporated.

- Adjust Sweetness:

  - Taste the mousse and adjust the sweetness according to your preference by adding more sweetener if needed.

- Chill:

  - Transfer the mousse to individual serving dishes or one large bowl.

  - Cover and refrigerate for at least 1-2 hours to chill and allow the flavors to meld.

- Serve:

  - Once chilled, you can serve the chocolate avocado mousse as is or top it with whipped cream, berries, or chopped nuts.

This low-carb chocolate avocado mousse is not only rich and satisfying but also packed with healthy fats and nutrients. The natural creaminess of avocados creates a silky texture, and the cocoa powder adds a rich chocolate flavor without the excess carbs. Enjoy this guilt-free dessert!

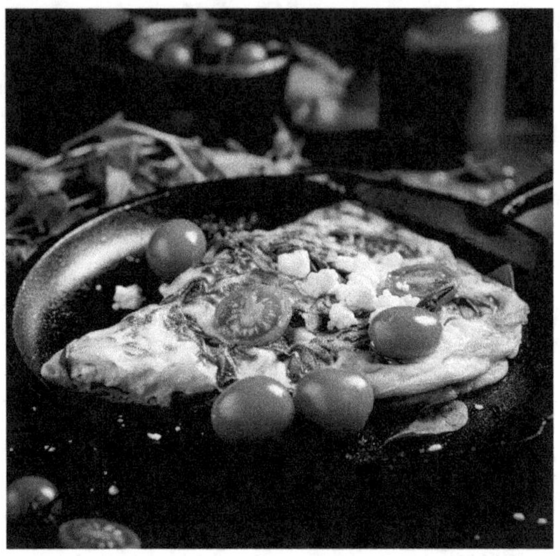

Low-Carb Spinach and Feta Omelet

Ingredients:

- 2 large eggs

- 1 cup fresh spinach, chopped

- 1/4 cup feta cheese, crumbled

- 1 tablespoon olive oil

- Salt and pepper to taste

- Optional: Cherry tomatoes, sliced avocado, or your favorite low-carb veggies for extra flavor

Instructions:

- Prep Ingredients:

  - Chop the fresh spinach and crumble the feta cheese.

- Whisk Eggs:

  - Crack the eggs into a bowl, add a pinch of salt and pepper, and whisk until well combined.

- Cook Spinach:

  - Heat olive oil in a non-stick skillet over medium heat.

  - Add chopped spinach and sauté for 1-2 minutes until wilted.

- Pour Eggs:

  - Pour the whisked eggs over the sautéed spinach in the skillet.

- Add Feta:

  - Sprinkle crumbled feta cheese evenly over the eggs.

- Cook the Omelette:

  - Allow the omelet to cook without stirring for a minute or until the edges start to set.

- Fold and Finish:

  - Gently lift the edges of the omelet with a spatula to check if the bottom is golden.

- Once the bottom is set, carefully fold the omelet in half.

- Serve:

  - Slide the omelet onto a plate and garnish with additional feta, cherry tomatoes, or sliced avocado if desired.

This low-carb spinach and feta omelet is quick to make, high in protein, and packed with nutrients. It's a perfect way to start your day with a satisfying and healthy breakfast! Feel free to customize it with your favorite low-carb veggies or herbs.

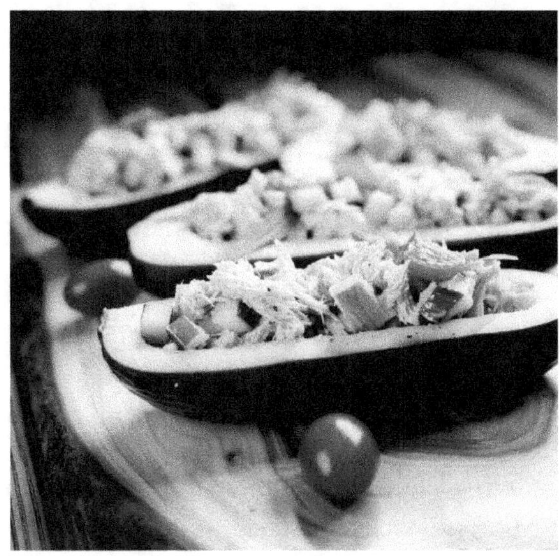

Low-Carb Avocado and Tuna Salad Stuffed Cucumber Boats

Ingredients:

- 1 large cucumber

- 1 ripe avocado

- 1 can (5 oz) tuna, drained

- 1 tablespoon mayonnaise

- 1 teaspoon Dijon mustard

- Salt and pepper to taste

- Optional: Fresh herbs like cilantro or chives for garnish

Instructions:

- Prepare the Cucumber Boats:

  - Wash the cucumber and cut it in half lengthwise. Scoop out the seeds to create "boats."

- Make the Tuna Salad:

  - In a bowl, mash the ripe avocado.

  - Add drained tuna, mayonnaise, Dijon mustard, salt, and pepper. Mix until well combined.

- Fill the Cucumber Boats:

  - Spoon the tuna and avocado mixture into the cucumber boats.

- Garnish:

  - Garnish with fresh herbs like cilantro or chives for added flavor.

- Serve:

  - Enjoy these refreshing avocado and tuna salad stuffed cucumber boats as a satisfying and low-carb snack!

This snack is not only delicious but also provides healthy fats and protein, making it a great option for a quick energy boost between meals. Feel free to adjust the ingredients based on your preferences.

Disclaimer

This book is intended to provide information and guidance on the topics discussed within its pages. However, readers are advised to exercise caution and discretion, as the content is not a substitute for professional medical advice, diagnosis, or treatment. The author is not a medical professional, and the information provided should not be considered a replacement for consultation with a qualified healthcare professional.

Possible Side Effects:

Individuals should be aware that implementing the suggestions and practices outlined in this book may have varying effects on different individuals. Side effects, both known and unknown, may occur. It is crucial to monitor your well-being and seek medical attention if any unexpected or adverse reactions arise.

Medical Supervision:

Some recommendations in this book may involve changes to lifestyle, diet, or exercise routines. Before making significant alterations, especially if you have pre-existing medical conditions, are pregnant, nursing, or taking medication, it is strongly advised to consult with a healthcare professional. Medical supervision ensures that any adjustments made align with your specific health needs and circumstances.

Assumption of Risk:

Readers must understand that they assume all risks associated with implementing the information provided in this book. The author and publisher shall not be held responsible for any outcomes resulting from the reader's application of the book's content.

In conclusion, while this book aims to empower and inform, readers are urged to prioritize their health and well-being. If in doubt, seek professional medical advice tailored to your circumstances.

Also By Mike Cunningham

- Happy by Choice: 50 Proven Ways to Achieve Lasting Happiness

- The Legends of Bluegrass: The Men and Women Who Created a Genre

- The Bride's Wedding Journal

- Word Search: Explore the Natural World

- Holiday Word Search

- Steam Punk City Coloring Book

- Mandalas Adult Coloring Book

- Relaxing Flowers Coloring Book

All are available on Amazon.com